RESEARCH REPORT

Factors Affecting Physician Professional Satisfaction and Their Implications for Patient Care, Health Systems, and Health Policy

The RAND Corporation

Mark W. Friedberg • *Peggy G. Chen* • *Kristin R. Van Busum* • *Frances M. Aunon*

Chau Pham • *John P. Caloyeras* • *Soeren Mattke* • *Emma Pitchforth*

Denise D. Quigley • *Robert H. Brook*

American Medical Association

F. Jay Crosson • *Michael Tutty*

Sponsored by the American Medical Association

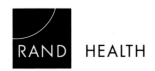

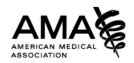

The research described in this report was sponsored by the American Medical Association, and was produced within RAND Health, a division of the RAND Corporation.

Library of Congress Cataloging-in-Publication Data is available for this publication.

ISBN 978-0-8330-8220-6

RAND OFFICES
SANTA MONICA, CA • WASHINGTON, DC
PITTSBURGH, PA • NEW ORLEANS, LA • JACKSON, MS • BOSTON, MA
DOHA, QA • CAMBRIDGE, UK • BRUSSELS, BE

Preface

The American Medical Association (AMA) has adopted, as a core strategic objective, the advancement of health care delivery and payment models that enable high-quality, affordable care and restore and preserve physician satisfaction. The AMA has undertaken this commitment in the belief that such change can and should result in a more sustainable and effective health care system with a highly motivated physician workforce. At the same time, the AMA has noted challenges for physicians interested in payment and delivery reform, including existing variability in the degree of care integration, the need for new skills and resources, and the uncertainty created by the emergence of as yet untested new payment models. Therefore, the AMA's objective includes facilitating transition, for physicians who are seeking a path to more integrated practice models, in a manner that supports professional satisfaction and practice sustainability. This objective is consistent with the mission of the AMA: To promote the art and science of medicine and the betterment of public health.

This project, sponsored by the AMA, aimed to characterize factors that influence physician professional satisfaction. By using a mixed-methods (primarily qualitative) design, the project sought to identify a broad array of potential targets for interventions to improve physician professional satisfaction. In accordance with the AMA's strategic objective and in the context of recent health reform legislation (including but not limited to the Affordable Care Act), changing fee-for-service payment rates, and perceived consolidation of independent physician practices by larger delivery systems, the influences of physician practice *model* (e.g., physician ownership versus hospital or other corporate ownership) and practice *sustainability* on professional satisfaction were of particularly high interest.

The project began on October 22, 2012, and was completed on September 30, 2013. An advisory committee convened by the AMA provided input on key study activities, including data collection methods and interpretation of results. Committee membership is listed in Appendix A.

Using project findings and input from other sources, including its membership and experts in physician practice design, the AMA plans to develop resources to assist physicians seeking to improve practice effectiveness, efficiency, sustainability, and professional satisfaction.

This work was sponsored by the American Medical Association. The research was conducted by RAND Health, a division of the RAND Corporation. A profile of RAND Health, abstracts of publications, and ordering information can be found at www.rand.org/health.

Contents

CHAPTER SIXTEEN

APPENDIXES

---

[1] Appendixes B through E can be found at http://www.rand.org/pubs/research_reports/RR439.html.

Figures

Tables

Executive Summary

Purpose

This project, sponsored by the American Medical Association (AMA), aimed to characterize factors that influence physician professional satisfaction. In the context of recent health reform legislation and other delivery system changes, we sought to identify high-priority determinants of professional satisfaction that can be targeted within a variety of practice types, especially as smaller and independent practices are purchased by or become affiliated with hospitals and larger delivery systems. Based on project findings and input from other sources, including its membership and experts in physician practice design, the AMA plans to develop possible pathways for American physicians to practice in models that are more effective, efficient, sustainable, and conducive to professional satisfaction.

Methods

Between January and August 2013, we gathered data from 30 physician practices in six states: Colorado, Massachusetts, North Carolina, Texas, Washington, and Wisconsin. We selected these practices to achieve diversity on practice size (<9 physicians, 10–49 physicians, >50 physicians), specialty (multispecialty, primary care, single subspecialty), and ownership model (physician owned or physician partnership, hospital or other corporate ownership). Although not designed to be nationally representative, this sampling strategy allowed inclusion of a broad swath of physician practice models and in-depth data collection from each. Each practice completed a structural questionnaire assessing its organizational structure, electronic health record use and capabilities, and participation in innovative payment models. We then visited each practice and conducted semistructured interviews with a total of 220 informants (108 with practicing physicians and 112 with practice leaders and other clinical staff), querying factors that influenced professional satisfaction within the practice, the local health care system, and the policy environment. Finally, we fielded a survey to 656 physicians in the 30 practices, receiving 447 responses (68-percent response rate). The survey used a combination of existing and new items to assess dimensions of professional satisfaction and factors that might influence professional satisfaction. We analyzed interview transcripts using qualitative software; identified common themes; and then, in the survey data, analyzed quantitative relationships corresponding to these qualitative themes.

Main Findings

We found that factors in several broad categories were important determinants of physician professional satisfaction, as detailed below. In our judgment, the most novel and important findings concerned how physicians' perceptions of quality of care and use of electronic health records affected professional satisfaction. The findings for quality and electronic health records (EHRs) were

- **Quality of care.** We found that, when physicians perceived themselves as providing high-quality care or their practices as facilitating their delivery of such care, they reported better professional satisfaction. Conversely, physicians described obstacles to providing high-quality care as major sources of professional dissatisfaction. These obstacles could originate within the practice (e.g., a practice leadership unsupportive of quality improvement ideas) or could be imposed by payers (e.g., payers that refused to cover necessary medical services).

  These findings suggest that, when physician dissatisfaction is attributable to perceptions of quality problems, such dissatisfaction could be viewed as a "canary in the coal mine" for the quality of care—assuming that physicians are correct in their perceptions. Interventions that address these quality concerns, simultaneously improving both the quality of care patients receive and physician professional satisfaction, should be attractive to multiple stakeholders.

- **Electronic health records.** EHRs had important effects on physician professional satisfaction, both positive and negative. In the practices we studied, physicians approved of EHRs in concept, describing better ability to remotely access patient information and improvements in quality of care. Physicians, practice leaders, and other staff also noted the potential of EHRs to further improve both patient care and professional satisfaction in the future, as EHR technology—especially user interfaces and health information exchange—improves.

  However, for many physicians, the current state of EHR technology significantly worsened professional satisfaction in multiple ways. Poor EHR usability, time-consuming data entry, interference with face-to-face patient care, inefficient and less fulfilling work content, inability to exchange health information between EHR products, and degradation of clinical documentation were prominent sources of professional dissatisfaction. Some of these problems were more prominent among senior physicians and those lacking scribes, transcriptionists, and other staff to support data entry or manage information flow. Physicians across the full range of specialties and practice models described other problems, including but not limited to frustrations with receiving template-generated notes (i.e., degradation of clinical documentation). In addition, EHRs have been more expensive than anticipated for some practices, threatening practice financial sustainability.

  Some practices reported taking steps to address the causes of physician dissatisfaction with EHRs. These steps were, most commonly, to allow multiple modes of data entry (including scribes and dictation with human transcriptionists) and to employ other staff members (e.g., flow managers) to help physicians focus their interactions with EHRs on activities truly requiring a physician's training.

In addition to quality and EHRs, we found factors influencing physician professional satisfaction in each area described below. In general, these findings agreed with earlier studies of physician professional satisfaction. These confirmatory findings, explored in detail in this study, demonstrate the persistent impact of these factors on physician professional satisfaction over time and through major changes in the U.S. health care system. The areas were

- **Autonomy and work control.** Greater physician autonomy and greater control over the pace and content of clinical work were both associated with better professional satisfaction. For some physicians, having a leadership or management role within the practice was a key way of achieving autonomy. However, practice ownership was not for everyone: Some physicians reported little taste for the "business side" of medicine, deriving satisfaction from employed positions that allowed them to focus more exclusively on clinical care.

  Because interviewees reported that practice structure and ownership could facilitate or limit their autonomy and ability to control their work, we also investigated the relationships between practice model and overall satisfaction. In our sample, physicians in physician-owned practices or partnerships were more likely to be satisfied than those in other ownership models (hospital or corporate ownership). However, we also found that strategies to enhance physicians' abilities to control the factors immediately affecting their day-to-day clinical work may be important to preserving or enhancing professional satisfaction within hospital- or corporate-owned practices.

- **Practice leadership.** Among the practices we studied, practice leadership affected physician professional satisfaction in two main ways. First, professional satisfaction was higher when physicians and their clinical colleagues reported that their values were well aligned with those of their leaders. Values alignment was especially important concerning approaches to clinical care. Some physicians reported that having leaders with clinical experience (either as physicians or other types of front-line clinical staff) enhanced the sense of values alignment between practice leaders and practicing physicians. Second, physicians reported better professional satisfaction when practice leadership took a balanced approach to new practice-wide initiatives, maintaining physician professional autonomy when possible.

- **Collegiality, fairness, and respect.** Physicians' perceptions of collegiality, fairness, and respect were key determinants of professional satisfaction. Physicians reported four main areas in which these constructs operated: relationships with colleagues in the practice (including practice leadership), relationships with providers outside the practice, relationships with patients, and relationships with payers. Within the practice, frequent meetings with other physicians and allied health professionals (such as business meetings in physician partnerships) fostered greater collegiality. Some physicians who no longer co-owned their practices observed that, when business meetings ceased, interpersonal familiarity with their former partners decreased, leading to lower overall morale.

  Physicians reported limited but important specialty-specific frustrations with unfairness and disrespect when interacting with other providers. For surgeons, these concerns surfaced most prominently in arranging hospital call duties. For primary care physicians, interactions with other physicians were problematic when primary care physicians (and their staffs) were treated as subservient.

- **Work quantity and pace.** Physicians, clinical staff, and practice leaders commonly reported challenges stemming from the quantity and pace of physician work. Especially in primary care specialties, physicians described how pressure to provide greater quantities of services effectively limited the time and attention they could spend with each individual patient, detracting from the quality of care in some cases. Some of the physicians we interviewed had joined practices in which payment did not rely on number of patients seen, but in doing so, they reported accepting lower incomes. Others reported that improvement strategies adapted from other industries (e.g., "lean" improvement techniques) had improved patient flow, making the pace of work more reasonable and reducing time pressures.

  Importantly, a smaller number of physicians and practices reported that dissatisfaction (and worries about practice sustainability) could also stem from insufficient work quantity. These concerns were most commonly articulated by the surgeons in our study.

- **Work content, allied health professionals, and support staff.** In general, physicians described better satisfaction when their work content matched their training and dissatisfaction when they were required to perform work that other staff could perform—especially when they sensed that the content of their work was being dictated to them. Specific types of satisfying work varied by specialty and by individual, but some patterns emerged. For example, many primary care physicians appreciated providing care that was continuous, including inpatient care. Some of these physicians missed caring for hospitalized patients, expressing concern about lost skills when hospitalists cared for their inpatients. Among surgeons, some expressed a desire to develop expertise in a specific niche within their field.

  Working with adequate numbers of well-trained, trusted, and capable allied health professionals and support staff was a key contributor to greater physician professional satisfaction. Support from such staff enabled physicians to achieve a more desirable mix of work content. Several study participants appreciated having long-term working relationships with allied health professionals and support staff, with some such relationships spanning decades. This theme was corroborated in quantitative analyses of physician survey responses, which revealed that greater staff stability (i.e., lower turnover) was a significant predictor of better overall professional satisfaction.

- **Payment, income, and practice finances.** Few physicians reported dissatisfaction with their current levels of income. However, physicians reported that income stability was an important contributor to overall professional satisfaction, and some described taking steps to preserve their incomes when pay rates decreased (or other changes threatened to reduce income). In addition, payment arrangements that were perceived as fair, transparent, and aligned with good patient care enhanced professional satisfaction. When practices changed their internal payment arrangements, clear and logical explanations for these changes were described as being important to preserving a sense of fairness. Physicians were less tolerant of income reductions that were perceived as resulting from the poor business decisions of practice leaders.

  Interviewees from practices of all specialties expressed a sense that relative incomes would shift in the future, with primary care gaining and some subspecialties potentially losing income. This was a source of concern for some subspecialist physicians and for practices that had invested heavily in subspecialty care. Worries about practice financial sustainability, when present, were described as a source of dissatisfaction. For some physicians, working in practices in which they did not have an ownership interest (e.g., working for a hospital-owned practice) alleviated the stress associated with ownership.

- **Regulatory and professional liability concerns.** Physicians and practice managers described the externally imposed rules and regulations under which they operated as having predominantly negative effects on professional satisfaction. Among these, "meaningful-use" rules stood out as having the greatest influence on professional satisfaction at the time of this study. While physicians agreed generally with the intent of meaningful-use rules, they expressed frustration with the time and documentation burdens these rules imposed—especially when they believed they were being asked to generate new documentation of activities that they had already performed.

  Professional liability concerns were not prominent contributors to dissatisfaction among the practices we sampled. As our interviews revealed, recent state-specific reforms to professional liability laws may have contributed to this finding. Had the study been conducted in other states, this finding could have been different.

- **Health reform.** Aside from incentives to adopt EHRs, our study did not identify recent health reforms as prominent contributors to overall physician professional satisfaction, either positively or negatively. In general, physicians and administrators expressed uncertainty about how various aspects of health reform (including but not limited to those contained in the Affordable Care Act) would affect physician professional satisfaction and practice financial sustainability. Leaders in multiple practices reported that transitions from one payment model (e.g., fee-for-service) to another (e.g., shared savings or capitation) would be complicated, with physicians receiving mixed incentives from different payers. In response to these concerns, several practices sought economic security by increasing their size or becoming affiliated with hospitals and large delivery systems. Leaders of smaller, independent practices that did not initiate such growth or affiliation described feeling pressure to join larger systems, sensing that it would become more difficult in the future to remain independent from these systems as a consequence of health reform.

Conclusions

Many of the factors influencing physician professional satisfaction identified in this study are shared by professionals and workers in a wide variety of settings. Therefore, the same considerations that apply outside medicine—for example, fair treatment; responsive leadership; attention to work quantity, content, and pace—can serve as targets for policymakers and health delivery systems that seek to improve physician professional satisfaction. This may seem an obvious conclusion, but considering the typical tools used to influence physician behavior (regulations, payment rules, financial incentives, public reporting, and the threat of legal action), refocusing attention on the targets identified in this study may actually represent a substantial change of orientation for many participants in the U.S. health care system.

EHR usability, however, represents a unique and vexing challenge to physician professional satisfaction. Few other service industries are exposed to universal and substantial incentives to adopt such a specific, highly regulated form of technology, one that our findings suggest has not yet matured. On one hand, only one in five physicians we surveyed would prefer to return to paper-based medical records. Nearly all physicians we interviewed saw the benefits of EHRs (e.g., remote accessibility to patient data) and believed in the "promise of EHRs." On the other hand, physicians cannot buy, install, and use a promise to help them deliver patient care. The current state of EHR technology appears to significantly worsen professional satisfaction for many physicians—sometimes in ways that raise concerns about effects on patient care.

Physicians look forward to future EHRs that will solve current problems of data entry, difficult user interfaces, and information overload. Specific steps to hasten these technological advances are beyond the scope of this report. However, as a general principle, our findings suggest including improved EHR usability among federal EHR certification criteria. In addition, the meaningful-use rules may not provide physicians with sufficient flexibility to match the needs of their practices—especially for those who do not provide primary care.

Finally, our finding that physicians are more satisfied when they perceive that they are meeting their patients' needs by delivering high-quality care—and dissatisfied when they perceive barriers to delivering high-quality care—suggests an additional way of thinking about the relationship between physician professional satisfaction and the quality of care that patients receive. Aside from viewing better patient care as a potential consequence of better physician professional satisfaction, it may be useful to think of physician dissatisfaction, when it is caused by perceived quality problems, as an indicator of potential delivery system dysfunction.

In this view, the critical step is to understand *why* some physicians report dissatisfaction with certain aspects of their professional lives. Some obstacles to professional satisfaction may have limited direct relationships to the quality of care. However, when dissatisfaction stems from factors that physicians perceive as compromising quality, further investigation of these factors may help identify important opportunities to improve patient care.

Put another way, producing a greater number of "satisfied" physicians is not the only goal. Even physicians who report high overall professional satisfaction will have sources of stress, frustration, and burnout in their clinical practices. Some of these stressors interfere with patient care. Solving them should be a high priority for multiple stakeholders.

Implications

This study raises important issues and questions to be addressed by researchers, policymakers, and health care leaders:

- **Physician practices need a knowledge base and resources for internal improvement.** In particular, many physician practices need help with managing change. Where will this come from? Larger physician practices have begun to apply such techniques as lean improvement with success, but for the majority of physician practices, such interventions are out of reach without help. Are hospitals and health systems the only sources of such practice improvement support?
- **As physician practices affiliate with large hospitals and health systems, paying attention to professional satisfaction may improve patient care and health system sustainability.** Consolidation of physician practices may improve or detract from physician satisfaction over the longer term. When dissatisfaction accompanies system consolidation, it will be important to understand the underlying causes: Does dissatisfaction stem from perceived barriers to delivering quality care, and if so, are these perceptions correct?

- **When implementing new and different payment methodologies, the predictability and perceived fairness of physician incomes will affect professional satisfaction.** Some but not all physicians and delivery systems seek alternatives to traditional fee-for-service payment, and transitions between payment models will be smoothest if incomes can be stabilized even as incentives change.
- **Better EHR usability should be an industrywide priority and a precondition for EHR certification.** Speeding the improvement of EHR usability may require direct incentives for EHR vendors. Until EHR usability improves dramatically, to the point that directly interacting with an EHR neither creates additional, excessive clerical work for physicians nor distracts from patient care, removing regulatory and legal barriers to using other practice staff (e.g., scribes) to interact directly with EHRs will allow physicians more time to perform work that requires physicians' training.
- **Reducing the cumulative burden of rules and regulations may improve professional satisfaction and enhance physicians' ability to focus on patient care.** Physicians reported feeling overwhelmed by the cumulative effect of rules and regulations on their ability to deliver patient care, especially when mandated activities (such as duplicative information entry) were perceived as a distraction from patient care. Reducing this burden in a responsible way will require cooperation between physician practices and both public and private sources of these rules and regulations.

Acknowledgments

The authors gratefully acknowledge the invaluable time, expertise, and knowledge generously contributed by leaders, physicians, and other staff in the 30 physician practices that participated in this study. The authors also gratefully acknowledge the efforts of leaders and staff members from the following state medical societies and associations, who facilitated practice participation in this study: the Colorado Medical Society, the Massachusetts Medical Society, the North Carolina Medical Society, the Texas Medical Association, the Washington State Medical Association, and the Wisconsin Medical Society.

In addition, the authors gratefully acknowledge the following individuals who provided input for this report: Eileen Rubey, American Medical Association; Kenneth Sharigian, American Medical Association; John E. Billi, University of Michigan Medical School; Lawrence Casalino, Weill Cornell Medical College; Carolyn Clancy, Agency for Healthcare Research and Quality; Thomas Curry, Washington State Medical Association; Edward Murphy, Tower-Brook Capital Partners and Virginia Tech Carilion School of Medicine; Rick Wesslund, BDC Advisors; Nicholas Wolter, Billings Clinic; Christine Sinsky, Medical Associates Clinic and Health Plans; Thomas Sinsky, Medical Associates Clinic and Health Plans; Susan Ridgely, RAND; Aaron Kofner, RAND; Samuel Hirshman, RAND; Shawna Beck-Sullivan, RAND; Robert Rudin, RAND; and Lori Uscher-Pines, RAND.

Abbreviations

ACO   accountable care organization

AMA   American Medical Association

CAT   computed axial tomography

CEO   chief executive officer

EHR   electronic health record

ER   emergency room

HMO   health maintenance organization

IMG   international medical graduate (a physician who received his or her medical degree outside the United States)

IT   information technology

MA   medical assistant

MEMO   Minimizing Error, Maximizing Outcomes (a previous scientific study)

P4P   pay-for-performance

PCMH   patient-centered medical home

USMG   U.S. medical graduate

CHAPTER ONE

Introduction

A core strategic objective of the American Medical Association (AMA) is the advancement of health care delivery and payment models that enable high-quality, affordable care and restore and preserve physician satisfaction. The AMA has undertaken this commitment in the belief that such change can and should result in a more sustainable and effective health care system with a highly motivated physician workforce. At the same time, the AMA has noted challenges for physicians interested in payment and delivery reform, including existing variability in the degree of care integration, the need for new skills and resources, and the uncertainty created by the emergence of as yet untested new payment models. Therefore, the AMA's objective includes facilitating transition, for physicians who are seeking a path to more integrated practice models, in a manner that supports professional satisfaction and practice sustainability. This objective is consistent with the mission of the AMA: To promote the art and science of medicine and the betterment of public health.

In light of these goals, the AMA asked RAND Health to explore the factors that influence physician professional satisfaction. To do this, we sought to identify a broad array of potential targets for interventions to improve physician professional satisfaction. We were particularly interested in the effects of recent health reform legislation (including but not limited to the Affordable Care Act), changing fee-for-service payment rates, and perceived consolidation of independent physician practices by larger delivery systems, the influences of physician practice *model* (e.g., physician ownership versus hospital or other corporate ownership) and practice *sustainability* on professional satisfaction.

Methodology

Between January and August 2013, we gathered data from 30 physician practices in six states: Colorado, Massachusetts, North Carolina, Texas, Washington, and Wisconsin. We selected these practices to achieve diversity on practice size (<9 physicians, 10–49 physicians, >50 physicians), specialty (multispecialty, primary care, single subspecialty), and ownership model (physician owned or physician partnership, hospital or other corporate ownership). Although not designed to be nationally representative, this sampling strategy allowed inclusion of a broad swath of physician practice models and in-depth data collection from each. Each practice completed a structural questionnaire assessing its organizational structure, electronic health record use and capabilities, and participation in innovative payment models. We then visited each practice and conducted semistructured interviews with a total of 220 informants (108 with practicing physicians and 112 with practice leaders and other clinical staff), querying factors that influenced professional satisfaction within the practice, the local health care system, and the policy environment. Finally, we fielded a survey to 656 physicians in the 30 practices, receiving 447 responses (68-percent response rate). The survey used a combination of existing and new items to assess dimensions of professional satisfaction and factors that might influence professional satisfaction. We analyzed interview transcripts using qualitative software; identified common themes; and then, in the survey data, analyzed quantitative relationships corresponding to these qualitative themes.

Organization of This Report

Chapter Two of this report describes our literature review. Chapter Three describes our methodology, while Chapter Four presents our conceptual model. Chapter Five describes our survey sample.

Chapters Six through Fifteen present the main findings of this study by topic area. Each of these chapters gives an overview of findings and then presents qualitative results with illustrative participant quotes. Results are organized by theme, with each theme representing a factor influencing physician professional satisfaction. Quantitative findings follow the qualitative findings. Each chapter concludes with a brief review of relationships between study findings and previously published research. The chapters are written so that they can be read independently and in any order. Because of the overlapping nature of the topics in this report, some findings appear in more than one chapter.

Chapter Sixteen offers our conclusions and recommendations.

Finally, a series of appendixes provides supplemental materials. Appendix A lists the members of our advisory committee. Appendixes B through E, which are available on the web page for this document (http://www.rand.org/pubs/research_reports/RR439.html), offer our interview guides, practice structural questionnaire, and survey instruments.

CHAPTER TWO

Background: Scan of the Literature on Physician Professional Satisfaction

Overview

To provide context for the current study, we sought to summarize existing literature on physician satisfaction. We identified several key studies that examined physician professional satisfaction by analyzing data from large, national surveys of physicians providing direct patient care, including the Robert Wood Johnson Young Physicians Study (Hadley and Mitchell, 1997), the Physician Worklife Study (Williams et al., 1999), the Women Physicians' Health Study (Frank et al., 1999), and the Community Tracking Study/Health Tracking Physician Survey (Kemper et al., 1996). Although survey instruments differed from study to study, specific questions assessing professional satisfaction were similar enough to allow reasonable comparison and synthesis of their findings.

In general, these studies have indicated that overall physician satisfaction is relatively high, with the percentage of physicians reporting satisfaction with their careers (measured by reporting being very satisfied or somewhat satisfied or by reporting strong agreement or agreement with statements regarding satisfaction) ranging from 79 to 84 percent (Chen et al., 2012; Frank et al., 1999; Landon et al., 2002). We also note that some other studies reported moderately lower levels of satisfaction, on the order of 69–71 percent, but these studies were not nationally representative (Lewis et al., 1993a; Movassaghi and Kindig, 1989). Surveys employing higher thresholds for measuring satisfaction (e.g., counting only those who report the highest possible levels of satisfaction as "satisfied") indicate that 38–43 percent of physicians report this more strict definition of satisfaction (Landon, Reschovsky and Blumenthal, 2003; Leigh et al., 2002). A recent study painting a more alarming picture of physician professional satisfaction had a response rate far too low to allow valid estimates of professional satisfaction among U.S. physicians (approximately 2 percent of physicians who were sent the survey responded to it) (The Physicians Foundation, 2012).

Although well-designed and well-executed surveys demonstrate that a minority of physicians report dissatisfaction with their careers, the persistence of this group may be cause for concern, especially if physician professional dissatisfaction reflects or contributes to problems in patient care.

Published studies have examined three general factors that influence physician professional satisfaction: physician demographics, workplace attributes, and factors related to the broader health care system. In addition, a significant body of work has investigated relationships between physician professional satisfaction and care patients received, including health outcomes. Below, we summarize the published literature in these areas.

Physician Demographics

Demographic characteristics—defined here as relatively immutable attributes, such as age, domestic versus foreign medical school, race/ethnicity, and specialty—have been shown to be associated with physician professional satisfaction.

Physician Age

Studies utilizing data from the Community Tracking Study/Health Tracking Physician Study have reported a U-shaped curve in the relationship between age and satisfaction, with younger physicians (<35 years) and older physicians (>65 years) reporting the highest levels of overall satisfaction and middle-aged physicians reporting lower satisfaction relative to those two groups (Leigh, Tancredi and Kravitz, 2009; Leigh et al., 2002). The authors propose two potential explanations for this finding: Younger physicians may be more idealistic, while physicians who have reached retirement age and have not yet left the practice of medicine are likely to be those who find greater enjoyment from their work.

Other work, utilizing the Physician Worklife Study but limiting the analysis to general internists, did not find this U-shaped curve but instead reported a monotonic relationship between age and satisfaction, with older physicians reporting greater satisfaction than younger physicians (Wetterneck et al., 2002). This finding was echoed in an analysis of the Women Physicians Study (Frank et al., 1999), a survey that included female physicians of all specialties. A possible explanation is that less-satisfied physicians tend to exit the profession, leaving a cohort of especially satisfied physicians who are still practicing in the oldest age groups.

Note that the difference in findings between the Community Tracking Study/Health Tracking Physician Study's U-shaped findings and the linear relationship of the Physician Worklife Study and the Women Physicians' Study report may be due to the way in which age was conceptualized. The analyses of Community Tracking Study/Health Tracking Physician Study data treated physician age as a categorical variable; in contrast, the Physician Worklife Study and the Women Physicians' Study treated age as a continuous variable.

Domestic Versus Foreign Medical School

Multiple analyses of data from the Community Tracking Study/Health Tracking Physician Survey have found that graduates of foreign medical schools report lower overall career satisfaction than graduates of U.S.-based medical schools (Boukus, Cassil and O'Malley, 2009; Chen et al., 2012; Landon et al., 2006; Leigh et al., 2002; Pagan, Balasubramanian, and Pauly, 2007; Stoddard et al., 2001). Outside the Community Tracking Study/Health Tracking Physician Study, international medical graduate status, in general, has not been included in studies examining physician satisfaction. The Women Physicians' Study did include birthplace (born inside versus outside the United States), with analyses demonstrating that U.S.-born physicians report slightly higher rates of satisfaction than their non–U.S.-born counterparts (Frank et al., 1999). However, it is important to caution that both these variables may be somewhat imprecise in their measurements. Using place of birth to identify international medical graduates would misclassify those who immigrated to the United States at an early age and attended U.S. medical schools as international medical graduates. Conversely, in addition, using country of education as a proxy for place of birth would misclassify U.S. citizens who go abroad for medical school as foreign-born physicians. Understanding the limitations to both these designations is important for interpreting these data.

Physician Race and Ethnicity

Existing studies report differing results regarding the relationship between race/ethnicity and overall career satisfaction. One relatively small study (but with a nationwide sample) of primary care physicians reported no statistical difference in professional satisfaction by race (Buchbinder et al., 1999; Buchbinder et al., 2001). However, the Women Physicians' Study reported that nonwhite physicians were more satisfied than white physicians, with Hispanic physicians reporting the highest levels of satisfaction, followed by physicians reporting black, other, and Asian race, respectively (Frank et al., 1999). Conversely, a study of Massachusetts physicians reported that white physicians were less likely than nonwhite physicians to report being dissatisfied with their practice situation (Quinn et al., 2009). A study of primary care physicians in the Seattle area reported similar findings, with white physicians being more likely than nonwhite physicians to report job satisfaction (Grembowski et al., 2003).

Physician Specialty

Existing studies vary widely in the specialties included for analysis. Generally, pediatricians have been found in a number of studies to report higher satisfaction than other specialties, while general internists have been found to report lower satisfaction than other specialties.

Analysis of data from the Community Tracking Study/Health Tracking Physician Survey, utilizing family medicine physicians as the referent group, indicate that pediatricians, geriatricians, dermatologists, and neonatologists were more likely to report overall job satisfaction, while otolaryngologists, obstetrician/gynecologists, ophthalmologists, orthopedic surgeons, and internists were less likely to report overall job satisfaction (Leigh et al., 2002). Geriatricians exhibited the greatest likelihood of reporting job satisfaction, while otolaryngologists had the greatest likelihood of reporting dissatisfaction. Other analyses from the Community Tracking Study/Health Tracking Physician Survey have found that after adjusting for covariates, pediatricians report greater job satisfaction than family medicine physicians, while general internists report less job satisfaction. In the same study, an examination of subspecialists indicates that obstetricians/gynecologists report less satisfaction than a referent group consisting of medical subspecialists (Stoddard et al., 2001). An analysis of more recent data from the Community Tracking Study/Health Tracking Physician Survey indicate that pediatricians are more likely than general internists to report career satisfaction (Chen et al., 2012). Additionally, one study of primary care physicians in the Seattle area indicated that family practitioners were more likely than general internists to report career satisfaction (Grembowski et al., 2003). Another study of primary care physicians in Massachusetts reported that general internists were the most dissatisfied group, in comparison with pediatricians, family medicine physicians, and subspecialists who practiced as primary care physicians (Landon et al., 2002).

Another study analyzing data from the Community Tracking Study/Health Tracking Physician Survey categorized specialties as "Controllable" (including dermatology; emergency medicine; neurology; ophthalmology; otolaryngology; and child, adolescent, and adult psychiatry) or "Uncontrollable" (including family practice, general practice, internal medicine, internal medicine and pediatrics–combined, obstetrics and gynecology, orthopedic surgery, pediatrics, general surgery, and urology), finding that being in an uncontrollable specialty was associated with lower career satisfaction (Leigh, Tancredi and Kravitz, 2009). The classification of specialties as controllable or uncontrollable was based on prior work, which identified a controllable specialty as one with a controllable lifestyle, largely defined as having control over work hours (Dorsey, Jarjoura and Rutecki, 2003).

Workplace Factors

Workplace factors—including practice structure (size, ownership, academic affiliation), geographic location, patient population, working environment (including autonomy and control over work), relationships with coworkers, perceived quality of patient care, electronic health records, and physician income—may have effects on physician satisfaction. Many, but not all, studies investigating these effects rely on evidence from large, nationally representative surveys of physicians.

Practice Structure

Studies utilizing data from the Community Tracking Study/Health Tracking Physician Survey report a significant relationship between practice size and likelihood of reporting career satisfaction; physicians in practices of one to two physicians generally reported lower satisfaction (Chen et al., 2012; Stoddard et al., 2001) and greater likelihood of leaving the practice within two years (Landon et al., 2006) than those in larger physician groups. These findings were also reported in analyses of data from the Physician Worklife Study (Linzer et al., 2000) and in a study utilizing data from one county in Arizona (Warren, Weitz and Kulis, 1998).

The results for how ownership structure affected physician satisfaction were mixed. While some studies utilizing Community Tracking Study/Health Tracking Physician Survey data from 2004–2005 indicate no statistically significant difference in satisfaction between physicians who were full or partial owners of their practices and those who were nonowners (Boukus, Cassil and O'Malley, 2009; Leigh, Tancredi and Kravitz, 2009), another study, using Community Tracking Study/Health Tracking Physician Survey data from 1998, found that physicians who were sole proprietors (full owners) were less likely than part or nonowner physicians to report being very satisfied (Leigh et al., 2002). This difference in results may reflect changes in the broader health care system that occurred in the approximately six years between surveys; these changes may have modified the effects of practice ownership on physician satisfaction.

Finally, a positive association between working in an academic environment and reporting career satisfaction has been reported in analyses of data from the Community Tracking Study/Health Tracking Physician Survey (Leigh, Tancredi and Kravitz, 2009; Pagan, Balasubramanian and Pauly, 2007; Stoddard et al., 2001). These data have also been used to demonstrate that physicians in medical school–based practices are less likely than those in other practice models to leave the practice within two years (Landon et al., 2006). Similar findings were reported in a national study of emergency physicians (Cydulka and Korte, 2008).

Geographic Location

Physicians practicing in rural locations generally reported high overall satisfaction compared with physicians in nonrural locations, as reported in analyses of data from the Women Physicians' Study (Frank et al., 1999), the Community Tracking Study/Health Tracking Physician Survey (Leigh et al., 2002), and a study of physicians in Massachusetts (Quinn et al., 2009). In addition, there may be differences in satisfaction levels among physicians classified as rural. One national study of physicians practicing in rural areas of the country (defined in the study as counties with populations of fewer than 1,000 individuals) reported that increased distance from a major referral center was associated with increased dissatisfaction (Movassaghi and Kindig, 1989).

Patient Population

Analyses of data from the Physician Worklife Study (Williams et al., 1999; Wetterneck et al., 2002) and a survey of primary care physicians in the Seattle area (Grembowski et al., 2003) indicated no statistically significant relationship between patient characteristics and physician satisfaction. However, data from the Community Tracking Study/Health Tracking Physician Survey indicated that physicians in communities with larger populations of uninsured patients were less likely to report career satisfaction (Pagan, Balasubramanian and Pauly, 2007).

Working Environment

In prior studies, physician professional satisfaction has been associated with physicians' perceptions of time pressure, control over their schedules, input into practice administration issues, and control over the content of their work.

Findings from a study of family practitioners and internists in New York and the Upper Midwest (An et al., 2009; Linzer et al., 2009), as well as from a study of academic and clinical faculty at one academic medical center (Linn, Yager, et al., 1985), indicated that greater time pressure to perform clinical duties was associated with lower physician satisfaction. A study of academic and clinical faculty at one academic medical center found associations between increased time spent supervising residents and increased day-to-day administrative responsibilities and lower professional satisfaction (Linn et al., 1986). Finally, a study of primary care physicians in Massachusetts reported that increased day-to-day administrative responsibilities were associated with lower physician satisfaction (Landon et al., 2002).

Physicians who reported higher levels of autonomy and control at work—as defined by questions querying control over work schedule, work content, and ability to make clinical decisions without outside interference—were also more likely to report greater satisfaction and lower rates of turnover. This relationship was found in a number of studies. One small national study of primary care physicians found that primary care physicians who had greater control over their work schedules were less likely to indicate that they planned to leave the practice within the next two years (Buchbinder et al., 2001). A study of physicians in Arizona found that physicians who felt a loss of control over work conditions and a decrease in clinical autonomy were more likely than those who did not feel these losses to report being dissatisfied (Warren, Weitz and Kulis, 1998). Data from the Community Tracking Study indicated that physicians who reported less control over the terms and content of their work and those who felt unable to provide needed services to patients were more likely to be dissatisfied with their careers in medicine than those who did not report these problems (Landon, Reschovsky and Blumenthal, 2003). Findings from the Physician Worklife Study indicated that physicians who reported less control in their workplaces were more likely to report stress than were colleagues who reported greater workplace control (Linzer et al., 2002). Similar findings have been reported among emergency physicians (Cydulka and Korte, 2008) and family practitioners and internists in New York and the Upper Midwest (Linzer et al., 2009).

Physicians' ability to choose which colleagues will receive their patient referrals has also been investigated as an aspect of autonomy and work control. Physicians who reported having the ability to make referrals to high-quality specialists were more likely than those who did not have this ability to report satisfaction, as reported in studies utilizing data from the Community Tracking Study/Health Tracking Physician Survey (Landon, Reschovsky and Blumenthal, 2003; Landon et al., 2006).

Relationships with Coworkers

Multiple studies with heterogeneous study populations have found that relationships with staff, colleagues, and practice managers and administrators have important effects on physician satisfaction. Those who perceived that practice managers and administrators valued and recognized their work were more likely to report career satisfaction than were those who perceived that their practice managers or administrators did not value and recognize their work. These findings were reported in studies utilizing data from a study of academic and clinical faculty at a single academic medical center (Linn, Yager, et al., 1985), a study of physicians in Texas (Lewis et al., 1993a), a study of family physicians in a single Midwest state (Karsh, Beasley and Brown, 2010), and a study of family practitioners and internists in New York and the Upper Midwest (Linzer et al., 2009).

Physicians who perceived good working relationships with other physicians (including perceptions of teamwork), as well as with staff in their practices, were also more likely to report being satisfied with their jobs and their overall career than were those who did not report good working relationships with other physicians. This was shown using data from the Physician Worklife Study (Williams et al., 1999; Linzer et al., 2000), the Community Tracking Study/Health Tracking Physician Survey (Stoddard et al., 2001), a study of academic and clinical faculty at a single academic medical center (Linn et al., 1986), a study of family physicians in a single Midwest state (Karsh, Beasley and Brown, 2010), a study of family practitioners and internists in New York and the Upper Midwest (Linzer et al., 2009), and a national study of emergency department physicians (Cydulka and Korte, 2008). Conversely, those who perceived insufficient support from colleagues and staff reported higher levels of dissatisfaction than did physicians who did report sufficient support from colleagues and staff (Lewis et al., 1993b).

Finally, those who perceived adequate opportunities for promotion or advancement in the practice reported great career satisfaction than did those who did not report having adequate opportunities, as evidenced by findings from a study of academic and clinical faculty at a single academic medical center (Linn et al., 1986) and a study of physicians in Texas (Lewis et al., 1993a).

Perceived Quality of Patient Care

Findings from the Physician Worklife Study indicated that perceived ability to deliver high-quality care to patients was positively associated with reporting satisfaction (Linzer et al., 2000). This finding was also reported in a study of academic and clinical faculty at one academic medical center (Linn, Brook, et al., 1985; Linn, Yager, et al., 1985).

Electronic Health Records

Although some physicians have used electronic health records (EHRs) for more than a decade, nationwide financial incentives to implement EHRs with certain functionalities are relatively new (stemming from the American Reinvestment and Recovery Act of 2009). As a result, the literature describing how EHRs affect physician satisfaction is sparse.

One study of physicians in Florida, based on a survey conducted in 2005, found that those who reported using an EHR and those who reported using a personal data assistant, such as a PalmPilot, were more likely to report satisfaction with both the level of computerization in their practice and with their current practice of medicine. This study also found that physicians who used email to communicate with their patients were less likely to report being satisfied with computerization in practice (Menachemi, Powers and Brooks, 2009). These seemingly discrepant findings are open to multiple interpretations. For example, it is possible that physicians who are early adopters of information technology, as indicated by their use of such devices as personal digital assistants, may have been be more likely to report being satisfied with the level of computerization in the practice and may also view the presence of an EHR as evidence of practice responsiveness to their preferences concerning information technology. However, those who communicate with patients via email may be dissatisfied with spending time on email without receiving payment for this work.

A survey of Massachusetts physicians conducted in 2005 found that those whose practice used EHRs were more likely to report dissatisfaction (Quinn et al., 2009). In a second survey of Massachusetts physicians conducted in 2007, 30 percent of physicians reported that their EHRs created new opportunities for error, but only 2 percent reported that their EHRs created more errors than they prevented (Love et al., 2012). In this 2007 survey, physician perception of new EHR-generated opportunities for error was associated with lower odds of reporting overall satisfaction with current practice. Finally, although applicability to the United States is unclear, a 2006 survey of physicians in Finland reported that stresses related to EHRs were associated with higher levels of overall stress and decreased productivity (Kuusio et al., 2012).

Physician Income

Higher income has been associated with greater professional satisfaction in a variety of studies, including the Women Physicians' Study (Frank et al., 1999), the Community Tracking Study/ Health Tracking Physician Survey (Boukus, Cassil and O'Malley, 2009; Leigh, Tancredi and Kravitz, 2009), a national study of emergency physicians (Cydulka and Korte, 2008), and a study of physicians in Texas (Lewis et al., 1993a). However, several studies utilizing data from the Community Tracking Study/Health Tracking Physician Survey indicated a slight drop in satisfaction among those in the highest income brackets, possibly indicating greater stress associated with maintaining very high levels of income (Chen et al., 2012; Leigh et al., 2002; Stoddard et al., 2001). Additionally, two studies utilizing data from the Physician Worklife Study (Wetterneck et al., 2002; Williams et al., 1999) found no association between income and physician satisfaction. However, both these studies were limited to general internists, and the within-specialty income variation may be too small to generate detectable effects.

In addition to absolute income, physicians' perceptions of earning "fair" incomes were some of the strongest indicators of overall satisfaction, as indicated in analyses of data from several studies, including a national study of physicians practicing in rural areas of the country (defined in the study as counties with populations of fewer than 1,000 individuals) (Movassaghi and Kindig, 1989), a study of academic and clinical faculty at a single academic medical center (Linn et al., 1986), and a study of physicians in Arizona (Warren, Weitz and Kulis, 1998).

Health System Changes

Changes in the broader health system (including but not limited to physicians' immediate workplaces) may also affect professional satisfaction. This is an important area of research given ongoing changes in the U.S. health care system. The Affordable Care Act has coincided with and, in many instances, spurred the growth of models of care delivery, such as patient-centered medical homes (PCMHs), accountable care organizations (ACOs), and other new models of care delivery and payment for care.

Although these innovations are too recent to have been extensively studied in the published literature, we report in this section on the existing evidence in potentially related areas, such as expansions in managed care and health maintenance organizations (HMOs) in the 1980s and 1990s. Some aspects of these past innovations may be relevant to the current changes in our health care system. For example, findings from past transitions to HMO models may foreshadow those that will emerge from participation in ACOs.

Managed care had mixed effects on physician satisfaction. Physicians in markets with larger proportions of managed care reported lower professional satisfaction in a variety of studies, including the Community Tracking Study/Health Tracking Physician Study (Leigh, Tancredi and Kravitz, 2009), a study of primary care physicians in Massachusetts (Landon et al., 2002), a study of primary care physicians younger than 45 years of age (Buchbinder et al., 2001), and a study of physicians in Arizona (Warren, Weitz and Kulis, 1998). This finding was especially pronounced among primary care physicians; a study utilizing earlier data from the Community Tracking Study/Health Tracking Physician Survey found that primary care physicians reported a significant decline in satisfaction associated with managed care, while the effect among specialists was not significant (Landon, Reschovsky and Blumenthal, 2003).

Although current PCMH models are relatively new (with multiple demonstrations currently under way), two studies indicated positive relationships between implementing a PCMH model, lower physician burnout, and better staff morale (Lewis et al., 2012; Reid et al., 2010). However, limitations of study design (one was a cross-sectional study, Lewis et al., 2012, and the other was in a single-practice site, Reid et al., 2010) leave much unknown about how PCMH transformation will affect professional satisfaction (Friedberg, 2012).

With regard to the legal and regulatory environment, one study utilizing data from the Physician Worklife Study reported that the "hassle factor" stemming from economic and regulatory forces external to the practice organization (e.g., insurance authorizations and gatekeeping requirements) was significantly and negatively correlated with satisfaction (Konrad et al., 1999).

Downstream Effects of Physician Professional Satisfaction

We also sought to examine the downstream effects of physician professional satisfaction or dissatisfaction on such dimensions as patient access to care, the overall physician workforce, physician retention, and health care costs.

While we found no published studies examining direct relationships between physician professional satisfaction and patient access to care, several studies did report a significant relationship between decreased physician satisfaction and greater workforce attrition, which could reduce the size of the available physician workforce. To better study workforce attrition, one national study surveyed primary care physicians younger than 45 years old at two points separated by three years to determine which physicians had left their original practices, finding that physicians who reported dissatisfaction in the first survey were more than twice as likely to leave their practices as those who did not report dissatisfaction (Buchbinder et al., 2001). Another study utilizing data in two rounds of the Community Tracking Study/Health Physician Tracking Survey compared physicians who reduced their work hours per week or left the practice of medicine between the first and second round of data collection. Those who reported greater dissatisfaction in the first data collection period were more likely to have left the practice of medicine or reduced their hours in the second data collection period (Landon et al., 2006). Finally, a study utilizing data from the Physician Worklife Survey examined reported intent to leave the practice within two years (Linzer et al., 2000) and found that dissatisfaction was strongly associated with reported intent to leave, although no data were available to determine whether physician job turnover actually occurred.

Physician satisfaction was not associated with the quality of care provided to patients in a study of family practitioners and general internists in New York and the upper Midwest (Linzer et al., 2009). However, in another small study of primary care physicians, patient adherence to medical treatment exhibited a positive association with physician satisfaction (DiMatteo et al., 1993). This study also reported a strong positive association between physician satisfaction and patient satisfaction, as did a number of other studies, including the study of clinical and academic faculty at a single academic medical center (Linn, Yager, et al., 1985), a study using both physician and patient data sets from the Community Tracking Study/Health Tracking Physician Study (DeVoe et al., 2007), and a study of general internists at academically affiliated practices in Massachusetts (Haas et al., 2000).

Finally, greater physician satisfaction has been associated with greater continuity of patient care. A study of clinical and academic faculty at a single academic medical center indicated that physicians who reported great satisfaction had lower no-show and cancellation rates, and patients had greater continuity of care as measured by the percentage of patients who saw the same provider on repeated visits (Linn, Brook, et al., 1985). Another study of primary care physicians in Seattle reported that patients with persistent pain were less likely to change physicians during a six-month follow-up period if they were seen initially by physicians who reported greater satisfaction with their jobs (Grembowski et al., 2005).

It is important to note that, because nearly all studies cited in this literature review have a cross-sectional design, it is not possible, in general, to determine the direction of causation when associations are identified. For example, relationships between physician professional satisfaction and the quality of care, when present, have three explanations that are indistinguishable in the data: Greater professional satisfaction could cause physicians to deliver better care; the delivery of better patient care could cause physicians to experience greater professional satisfaction; or some unobserved third factor could cause both better patient care and greater professional satisfaction (creating an association without causation in either direction).

Summary

Broadly speaking, factors that influence physician satisfaction can be divided into three key categories: physician demographics, workplace factors, and changes in the health care system. Prior studies have demonstrated strong associations between physician satisfaction and certain factors including income, autonomy and work control, physician turnover, and patient satisfaction. The evidence linking newer developments, such as EHRs, PCMHs, and ACOs, to physician professional satisfaction is relatively scant.

The findings reviewed here helped guide the content and scope of data collection in the current study. Moreover, these findings give important context to our findings. Where relevant, we have pointed out relationships between our findings and the prior literature in each section presenting study results.

CHAPTER THREE

Methods

Overview of Methodological Approach

The project employed a mixed methods design, incorporating a primary qualitative component (multiple case studies, with each of 30 physician practices constituting a "case") and embedding a quantitative component to further investigate qualitative themes. We thus prioritized qualitative methods in the study design. While this prioritization required some sacrifices in quantitative design—for example, we conducted a physician survey within the study practices, rather than in a nationally representative sample—we preserved other aspects of quantitative rigor (e.g., achieving a high survey response rate, conducting appropriate statistical tests) to perform valid quantitative analyses within the study sample.

The project incorporated an emergent design, with periodic input on data collection methods and interpretation of results from the project advisory committee. Critical design decisions (such as the content of the physician survey and the codebook for qualitative analysis) were thus made during the project rather than fixed in advance. This design allowed us to explore unanticipated but important factors affecting physician professional satisfaction in depth as they emerged from the data collection and preliminary analyses.

Our overall methodological approach is summarized in Table 3.1 and discussed in more detail in the text that follows.

Justification for Mixed Methods

We chose a mixed-methods design to allow detection, via open-ended interview questions, of unanticipated factors influencing physician professional satisfaction while retaining the ability,

Table 3.1
Overview of Methodology

Strategy	Sample	Goal	Analysis
Semistructured interviews	Purposive: leaders, physicians, and other clinical staff in each of 30 practices	Identify factors influencing physician professional satisfaction	Qualitative coding of interview transcripts
Practice structural questionnaire	One questionnaire completed by the leadership of each practices	Measure aspects of practice structure (e.g., use of EHRs, payment models)	Context for qualitative analysis; multivariate regression models
Physician survey	Complete census or random sample (in large practices) of physicians within each practice	Assess individual physician professional satisfaction and correlates	Multivariate regression models

via analysis of written survey responses, to determine whether these influences were shared by a broader population of physicians than those we interviewed and to investigate factors that individual interviewees may have had limited ability to report from their own personal experiences (such as the influence of age or specialty on professional satisfaction).

This design was intended to address two potential shortcomings of the qualitative component alone. First, as described in more detail below, participants in the semistructured interviews were identified by practice leaders and therefore could represent viewpoints congruent with those of the leadership rather than those of the practice as a whole. Our physician survey addressed this concern by employing a sampling design that was reflective of all physicians within each practice. Second, due to the nature of physician careers, individual interviewees could not report, based on their own experiences, how certain factors of interest (such as practicing in a different specialty) would affect their professional satisfaction. Therefore, we investigated the relationships between specialty, clinical income (adjusted for work hours), and professional satisfaction, even though we did not ask qualitative interviewees to estimate on how hypothetical changes to their specialties or incomes would affect their professional satisfaction.

Data Collection

Overview

The project gathered qualitative and quantitative data from 30 participating physician practices between January and August 2013. We collected these data with the primary goal of conducting analyses to describe how factors at multiple levels (health system, organization, and individual physician) affect professional satisfaction. By creating a nested data structure of clinicians within sites and sites within practices, we aimed to explore how factors at these multiple levels interacted to affect these study outcomes.

Qualitative and quantitative data were collected concurrently, although for most practices, this occurred in the following sequence: first, the practice structural questionnaire; second, the semistructured interviews; and third, the physician survey.

This research project received an Adult Surveys and Interviews exemption from RAND's Human Subjects Protection Committee. Participants in all data collection activities gave informed consent to participate in this research.

Practice Sample

Because the factors influencing professional satisfaction and practice sustainability may vary by geographic location and by practice model, we purposively selected 30 practices to achieve diversity on the following observable dimensions:

- primary criterion: state
- secondary criteria: practice model
  - size (<9 physicians, 10–49 physicians, >50 physicians)
  - specialty (multispecialty, primary care, single subspecialty)
  - ownership model (physician owned or physician partnership, hospital or other corporate ownership).

These 30 practices were located in six states (five per state) selected for geographic diversity: Colorado, Massachusetts, North Carolina, Texas, Washington, and Wisconsin. While this sampling design did not generate a nationally representative group of all physicians or practices in the United States, it allowed inclusion of a broad swath of physician practice models and in-depth data collection from each, thus allowing reasonable generalizability of the findings.

In consultation with each state's medical society, we developed a list of practices for potential inclusion in the study. After gathering initial information on each potential practice's size, specialty, and ownership model, we invited selected practices to participate until five participants per state were identified, aiming for diversity on each practice design dimension within the state. The majority of practices invited agreed to participate, and those that declined cited competing organizational demands on time that made participation impractical. Among those agreeing to participate, all but one completed the study. This practice, which withdrew before data collection began (due to competing demands on practice leadership), was replaced by another practice in the same state.

Neither membership in the AMA nor in the corresponding state medical society was required for potential inclusion, and approximately 20 percent of physicians in the survey sample frame were AMA members at the time of the study (similar to national AMA membership rates). Because data collection required time commitments from practice leadership, physicians, and staff, it is also possible that truly struggling practices (i.e., those lacking the bandwidth for study participation) were underrepresented.

Tables 3.2 and 3.3 describe the final practice sample.

As shown in Table 3.3, we succeeded in sampling five practices from each state (the primary criterion). We achieved adequate representation of each structural dimension (the secondary criteria) as shown in Table 3.2. However, we were unable to sample practices with every *combination* of structural dimensions (as represented by the empty cells in Table 3.3). In general, the empty cells represent combinations of characteristics that are relatively rare in the United States (e.g., small multispecialty groups, large groups with just one specialty).

It is important to note that, due to the limited number of practices in each of the individual cells in Table 3.3, these interactions represented by the cells are not the main structural

Table 3.2
Final Practice Sample: Summary by Practice Model

	Category	Number of practices
Size	Large (>50 physicians)	9
	Medium (10–49 physicians)	11
	Small (<9 physicians)	10
Specialty	Multispecialty	15
	Primary care	10
	Single subspecialty	5
Ownership model	Physician-owned or partnership	19
	Hospital or corporate owner	11

Table 3.3
Final Practice Sample: Detailed State and Model Interactions

Size (number of physicians)	Physician-Owned or Partnership			Hospital or Corporate Owner		
	Multispecialty	Primary Care	Single Subspecialty	Multispecialty	Primary Care	Single Subspecialty
Large (>50)	NC-1 TX-2 TX-4			MA-1; MA-2 WA-3; WI-1 WI-2; WI-3		
Medium (10–49)	CO-3 WA-4 NC-5	WI-4	CO-4 NC-2	WI-5 MA-5 NC-4	WA-1	CO-1
Small (<9)		TX-1; TX-3 CO-2; CO-5 MA-3; MA-4 NC-3	TX-5 WA-5		WA-2	

analytic variables for this study. Instead, the practice structural dimensions in Table 3.2 are the structural analytic variables of interest. For example, we do not compare "small, physician-owned, primary care practices" to "large, hospital-owned, multispecialty" practices. Rather, we make comparisons on each dimension separately (for example, small versus large practices and physician versus hospital ownership).

Some of the practices had more than one site (i.e., more than one street address or building in which physicians provided care). Within the 30 practices included in the study, we collected data from 53 such sites.

Qualitative Data Collection: Semistructured Interviews During Site Visits

We visited each of the 30 participating practices between January and August 2013. Within each practice having multiple sites (e.g., large multispecialty practices), we visited two to four sites. To select these sites, we worked with practice leaders to identify a sample that would represent the typical range of physician experiences within the practice, including multiple specialties when possible.

During each site visit, a team consisting of a physician interviewer and at least one note taker conducted semistructured interviews with approximately four to six individuals per site (including practicing physicians, nonphysician clinicians, operational leadership, and financial/business leadership), yielding up to 18 interviews from practices with three to four sites. Most interviews were with individuals, but to accommodate respondent schedules, some were with groups of interviewees. We performed the majority of interviews on site to facilitate subject recruitment and to make notes on interpersonal dynamics, site physical layout, and other impressions of each practice (e.g., how busy the site seemed to be); we did not observe patient care directly. In all but the smallest practices (in which we interviewed all personnel), interviewees were selected by practice leadership; we had asked them to select interviewees who could describe an array of different experiences (e.g., senior physicians and those who had recently joined the practices). In cases of schedule conflict or new recommendations for interviewees, we conducted additional interviews via telephone after the site visits. With respondent consent, we recorded each interview.

To conduct the semistructured interviews, we developed guides for each type of respondent: practicing physicians, nonphysician clinicians, operational leadership, and financial or business leadership. We developed the guides based on a review of published literature on factors influencing physician professional satisfaction and with an intent to capture newer potential influences on professional satisfaction (e.g., new payment and organizational models, EHRs). These interview guides included questions intended to open discussion in several categories, such as work content, practice operations, recent changes to the practice, and how these changes affected professional satisfaction. As appropriate to semistructured interviews, interviewers followed respondents' leads, allowing the breadth and sequence of topics to flow naturally from respondents' answers to questions opening each topic. Each interview lasted 45 to 60 minutes and was transcribed for qualitative analysis. Between visits to the first six practices (one per state), we iteratively revised the interview guides to improve item clarity and interview flow. The final interview guides are available online, in Appendix B.

In total, we performed 220 semistructured interviews, including 108 interviews with physicians.

Quantitative Data Collection
Practice Structural Questionnaire

To characterize each of the participating practices, we developed a practice structural questionnaire to collect information on practice organization and staffing levels, patient volume and population demographics, enhanced access options, participation in innovative payment models, EHR capabilities, payer mix, physician compensation models, and financial position. This questionnaire was derived from earlier instruments developed by study staff and, with permission, financial questionnaires from the Medical Group Management Association (MGMA) (Friedberg et al., 2009). The questionnaire is available online, in Appendix C.

We sent the structural questionnaire to an administrative leader of each practice. To complete the questionnaire, each leader could enlist the help of other practice staff as necessary.

Physician Experience Survey

To gather data on physicians' professional satisfaction and factors potentially influencing professional satisfaction, we developed a pilot written survey instrument based on existing surveys of physician work experiences and input from the project advisory committee. This pilot instrument included items from previously validated scales to measure the following domains: global work satisfaction, stress, burnout, intent to leave, work control, chaos, time pressure, values alignment with leadership, adequacy of equipment and resources, satisfaction with income, patient care issues, and autonomy (from the Minimizing Error, Maximizing Outcomes [MEMO] study and Physician Worklife Study II, Linzer et al., 2009); pressure to attract and retain patients, receipt of quality and registry data, and compensation structure (from the Health Tracking Professional Survey, Center for Studying Health System Change, 2013); the relationship infrastructure, facilitative leadership, and sensemaking subscales of adaptive reserve (from the TransforMed Clinician and Staff Questionnaire, Jaen et al., 2010); and coordination of care (from the Safety Net Medical Home survey, Lewis et al., 2012). We edited some of these preexisting items to improve clarity and consistency of response tasks throughout the survey instrument.

We also developed new item sets to measure the quantity and content of clinical work, attitudes toward performance feedback received from the practice, perceptions of being respected as a professional, availability of allied health professionals and support staff, satisfaction with vacation and benefits, professional liability concerns and experience, and total income from clinical activities in the past year. Finally, the survey requested each respondent's age, gender, and other demographic characteristics.

After piloting the physician experience survey in the first six practices we visited (one per state), we added two additional types of items:

1. **EHR items.** Semistructured interviews during the pilot period revealed an unanticipated, recurring theme: Respondents reported that their EHRs had important effects on their professional satisfaction. The prior surveys from which we drew items were developed prior to nationwide financial incentives to adopt EHRs and did not include items specific to clinician experiences with EHRs. Therefore, we added two items assessing EHRs from the MEMO study (Linzer et al., 2009) and a longer set of original items querying specific themes encountered during qualitative interviews. These included EHRs' perceived effect on quality of care, speed of care, quality of communication with patients, work content, volume of clinical messages, and overall job satisfaction.

2. **Response tendency items.** From our review of the literature, we became concerned that observed associations between survey responses could result from variation in the response tendencies among individuals completing the survey. That is, inherently optimistic individuals would be expected to report greater professional satisfaction and higher ratings of many aspects of their practices (e.g., better relationships with practice leaders), and inherently pessimistic individuals would be expected to give opposing responses. This individual-to-individual variability in inherent optimism or pessimism (i.e., "response tendency") could generate spurious results in cross-sectional analyses of relationships between professional satisfaction and aspects of the practice environment. To address this threat to validity (a subtype of "common method bias"), we added two scales intended to measure the response tendency of each respondent directly, without reference to clinical activities or the practice environment (i.e., we attempted to construct "marker variables" that could be used to control for individuals' response tendencies) (Podsakoff et al., 2003):

   a. the Life Orientation Test–Revised (LOT-R), a scale that was developed to assess individual-to-individual variation in generalized optimism or pessimism (Scheier, Carver and Bridges, 1994)

   b. an original item set that asked respondents to rate a relatively uniform "common experience" to which all were likely to have been exposed (e.g., experiences with airport security screenings).

To field the survey, we obtained from each practice a list of all physicians who provided patient care at least one day per week in the practice at the time of data collection. We aimed to sample an average of 25 to 30 respondents per practice. To reach this average, we estimated the available sample sizes for each practice (before actually receiving sample frames) and drew samples as follows: If there were fewer than 70 eligible physicians within a given practice (within the sites we visited, if there were multiple sites), we sampled all eligible physicians. If there were more than 70 eligible respondents within the sites we visited, we sampled 70 respondents at random.

We sent an initial survey packet via first class mail to each sampled eligible respondent. Each survey packet included a letter of introduction, a letter of support from the AMA, the survey instrument, and a postage-paid return envelope. Nonrespondents received reminders via phone or email, as well as up to three remailings of the survey packet. Each respondent was offered an honorarium of $40 for completing the survey.

The final physician experience survey instrument is available online, in Appendix D.

Data Analysis

Overview

Our primary approach to integrating qualitative and quantitative data was, first, to identify qualitative findings and, second, to pursue quantitative analyses that followed threads from the qualitative interviews (O'Cathain, Murphy and Nicholl, 2010; Moran-Ellis et al., 2006). For example, if qualitative analysis of interview transcripts suggested that working with adequate numbers of allied health professionals and support staff produced better professional satisfaction, we would then follow that thread by quantitatively analyzing (from survey response data) the relationships between professional satisfaction, physicians' perceptions of whether there were enough allied health professionals and support staff in their practices, and the reported number of allied health professionals and support staff at each practice.

In addition to following themes from the qualitative interviews, we performed a limited number of supplemental quantitative analyses investigating factors that we believed could affect professional satisfaction and practice sustainability but that were not addressed directly in the interviews. We based these analyses on the conceptual model described below and on input from the advisory committee. In general, these supplemental quantitative analyses were suited to detecting relationships by making comparisons across individuals, rather than asking how a given change would affect a single interviewee. For example, we investigated the relationships between specialty, clinical income (adjusted for work hours), and professional satisfaction, even though we did not ask qualitative interviewees to estimate how hypothetical changes to their specialties or incomes would affect their professional satisfaction.

Theory Refinement: Developing a Conceptual Model

Working from previously published conceptual models of physician professional satisfaction (most notably, the conceptual model employed in the MEMO study [Linzer et al., 2009]) and input from the project advisory committee, we developed an initial conceptual model to represent possible relationships between three categories of conceptual inputs (health system context, practice organizational features, and physician individual characteristics), two products of interactions between these inputs (work characteristics and work perceptions), and three types of outcomes of these inputs and their interactions (physician outcomes, organizational outcomes, and patient outcomes).

We then updated the initial conceptual model, focusing on the specific items within each category, based on weekly research team discussions about the data obtained from each site visit. Each time a new emerging theme was identified, we attempted to place it within the model.

Qualitative Analyses

A seven-person multidisciplinary team, including a general internist, a general pediatrician, and five policy researchers, each with training and expertise in qualitative methods and health service research, performed the qualitative analyses. Five of the seven members of the data analysis team also performed site visits and conducted the semistructured interviews and therefore were familiar with the data. All qualitative coding was performed before any quantitative analyses were conducted.

The team developed a code structure using systematic, inductive procedures to generate insights grounded in the views the study participants had expressed (Bradley, Curry and Devers, 2007). To do this, the qualitative analysis team met weekly throughout the project to discuss each site visit, update the conceptual model, and expand or refine a running list of themes gathered from each practice visited. This list of themes, grouped by conceptual category, served as the initial codebook for qualitative analysis. Then, after nearly all interviews had been completed, the team coded the interview transcripts, using the constant comparative method to ensure that themes were consistently classified, while allowing expansion of existing codes, identification of novel concepts, and refinement of codes (Bradley, Curry and Devers, 2007). The qualitative analysis team used essential components of consensual qualitative research to code the interview transcripts, including consensually agreeing on the meaning of the data and auditing the work of each qualitative coder to ensure consistency (Hill et al., 2005; Kvale, 1996). Specifically, each member of coding team coded a set of interview transcripts independently. The two physician members of the coding team cross-checked each other's coding to ensure a common coding approach, then checked the work of the other coders. Any coder could suggest new codes for inclusion in the codebook; codebook additions or refinements were discussed by the full qualitative analysis team and decided by consensus.

We used Dedoose Version 4.5 (SocioCultural Research Consultants LLC, Los Angeles) to manage and analyze qualitative data.

Quantitative Analyses

For each clinician experience survey item, we calculated univariate response frequencies and descriptive statistics to assess item performance. Based on each respondent's specialty, we excluded nonapplicable items from analysis (e.g., items specific to office-based care were not applicable to hospitalists). After these exclusions, item nonresponse rates were less than 5 percent for all but one survey item: The item querying clinical income on the prior year had a nonresponse rate of 15 percent. Responses to quantitative items were in realistic ranges.

When survey items were drawn from a preexisting scale, we calculated scale scores based on the methods the scale developers used. In some cases, our survey revised these scales by adding or subtracting items, and we used parallel methods to calculate scores for these revised scales. For some original items new to the clinician experience survey, we created new scales and calculated the internal consistency of each. Methods for calculating each scale featured in the quantitative analyses are available in the annotated physician survey online, in Appendix E.

Nearly all survey items were included in both the pilot sample (six practices) and main sample (24 practices); survey responses to these items were pooled across these samples. By necessity, the survey items that were newly introduced in the main sample are analyzed within the main sample only (e.g., the items about EHRs).

We linked data from the practice structural questionnaires (including data on practice size, specialty, and ownership) and clinician experience surveys. When clinician experience survey items reflected practice-level constructs (e.g., practice culture), we aggregated responses within the practice by taking the within-practice mean. For example, we investigated associations between professional satisfaction and scores on the scale "Values Alignment with Leadership" at the individual physician level (which may reflect individual perceptions as much as characteristics of leaders) *and* at the practice level (which may more effectively isolate the influence of practice leaders by averaging out variations in individual-to-individual perceptions within a practice).

Then, for each theme emerging from the qualitative analyses, we constructed parallel quantitative analyses. For example, EHRs emerged from the qualitative analyses as an important factor influencing professional satisfaction, so we assessed quantitative relationships between EHR ratings and overall professional satisfaction in the clinician survey response data, using categorical and continuous statistical tests as appropriate. Physician "overall professional satisfaction" was the primary outcome in all quantitative analyses. However, we also analyzed related outcomes (burnout, stress, intent to leave practice, and intent to leave profession), finding similar relationships to the main analyses. For example, factors that increased the likelihood of reporting high overall professional satisfaction also lowered the risk of burnout.

Where conceptually appropriate, we adjusted or stratified survey responses to account for confounders. For example, we adjusted clinical income for hours worked per year by calculating an effective hourly wage. We also used multivariate regression to control for response tendency, and we used generalized estimating equations with empirical standard error estimates to account for clustering of observations within practices (Liang and Zeger, 1986; Zeger and Liang, 1986).

We considered P values <0.05 to be statistically significant. We managed and analyzed quantitative data using SAS 9.2 (SAS Institute Inc., Cary, NC).

Limitations of Study Methods

Both the qualitative and quantitative methods in this study had limitations. In the qualitative interviews, responses could have been subject to social desirability bias, in which interviewees may have given answers that they felt would be more "socially acceptable" than their true beliefs. For example, interviewees could have underreported income as a driver of their own professional satisfaction. The quantitative survey was intended, in part, to address this limitation, since the vast majority of items (especially those concerning sensitive topics, such as income) did not ask individual survey respondents to describe how specific factors affected their professional satisfaction. Instead, quantitative associations were inferred by combining responses from multiple survey respondents. In addition, our analysis of survey responses, which controlled for measures of individual response tendency, was designed to mitigate bias due to respondent-to-respondent variability in susceptibility to social desirability.

The major limitation of the quantitative survey was its lack of national representativeness. Therefore, survey responses could not be used to generate estimates of physician sentiment nationwide. In addition, despite assurances and fielding protocols specifically designed to protect the privacy and confidentiality of survey responses, some survey respondents may have altered their responses to some survey items out of concern that practice leaders would see their responses in a manner that would identify them or would enable deduction of their identities. Nonresponse analysis revealed that, despite obtaining a high overall survey response rate, the characteristics of survey respondents were not identical to nonrespondents on every measureable dimension.

CHAPTER FOUR

Conceptual Model

Like the initial conceptual model that guided data collection efforts, the final model that incorporated study findings represented possible relationships between three categories of conceptual inputs (health system context, practice organizational features, and physician individual characteristics), two products of interactions between these inputs (work characteristics and work perceptions), and three types of outcomes of these inputs and their interactions (physician outcomes, organizational outcomes, and patient outcomes).

In the final model (see Figure 4.1), the key physician outcomes were overall professional satisfaction, stress, burnout, intent to leave the practice or the profession, and physician health. The key organizational outcomes were practice sustainment, change, or disbandment and whether models of care (i.e., entire categories of practice design) succeed or fail. The specific patient outcomes were patient health, patient experience of care, access to care, and costs of care.

The conceptual model does not assume specific, directional relationships between the physician, organizational, and patient outcomes. Improvements in physician professional satisfaction could be accompanied by positive, negative, or no changes in organizational and patient outcomes. In the model, *the relationships between changes in physician, organizational, and patient outcomes depend on the reasons underlying these changes* (i.e., the upstream changes in inputs and their interactions). For example, a new policy requiring last-minute patients to see a dedicated urgent care provider could improve professional satisfaction (by alleviating the time pressure the patient's usual physician feels under a rigid scheduling model) but detract from patient outcomes if patients would prefer to see only their usual physicians. On the other hand, if a practice reengineers its workflows to accommodate last-minute appointments with patients' usual physicians (or more time to see unusually complex patients), both physician professional satisfaction and patient outcomes would be likely to improve. Interventions (i.e., changes to conceptual model inputs) that produce improvements in all three outcome categories would therefore be attractive to a broad array of stakeholders.

Figure 4.1
Final Conceptual Model

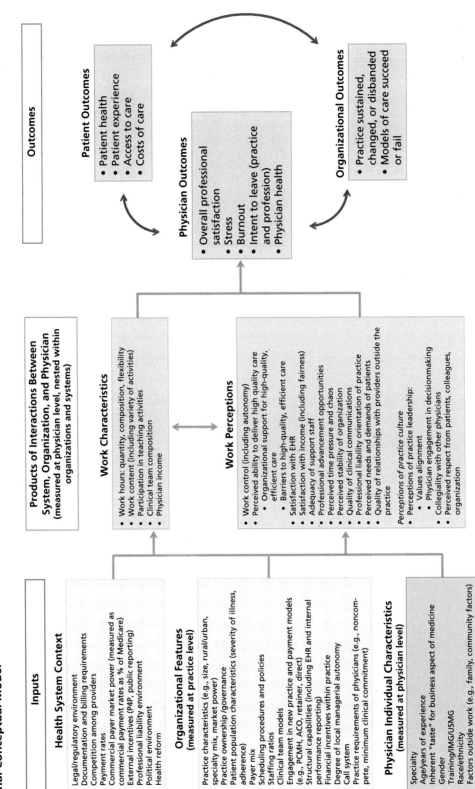

RAND RR439-4.1

CHAPTER FIVE

Characteristics of the Survey Sample

During the course of the study, we distributed 656 physician experience surveys, receiving a total of 447 responses (68-percent response rate). Table 5.1 presents nonresponse analyses,

Table 5.1
Characteristics of Respondents and Nonrespondents

Variable	Value	Respondents	Nonrespondents	P for Difference[a]
State	Colorado	12%	12%	0.04
	Massachusetts	22%	14%	
	North Carolina	16%	17%	
	Texas	15%	19%	
	Washington	14%	10%	
	Wisconsin	21%	27%	
Gender	Female	39%	41%	0.68
AMA membership	Current member	18%	15%	0.07
Age	Mean age	49 years	50 years	0.65
Individual physician specialty	Primary care	60%	48%	0.007
	Surgery and surgical subspecialty	15%	23%	
	Medical subspecialty	26%	29%	
Practice size	Small (<9 physicians)	6%	1%	0.003
	Medium (10–49 physicians)	44%	38%	
	Large (>50 physicians)	50%	60%	
Practice specialty	Multispecialty	76%	84%	0.02
	Primary care	8%	3%	
	Single subspecialty	15%	13%	
Practice ownership	Physician-owned or partnership	46%	49%	0.50
	Hospital or corporate owner	54%	51%	

[a] P values from Pearson Chi square tests for categorical variables (percentages) and Wilcoxon rank-sum tests for continuous variables (means). Individual physician descriptors are from the AMA Physician Masterfile, and practice-level characteristics were obtained during the study.

based on data available for both survey respondents and nonrespondents. Respondents were statistically significantly more likely than nonrespondents to be from Massachusetts and Washington, to specialize in primary care, to be in small or medium-sized practices, and to practice in primary care practices. There were no statistically significant differences by gender, AMA membership status, age, or practice ownership.

It is important to note that the survey sample in this study is *not* nationally representative. However, to provide context for the qualitative and quantitative findings in subsequent chapters, we present in Table 5.2 the overall rates of professional satisfaction and related constructs (stress, burnout, and intent to leave) among the survey respondents.

Table 5.2
Overall Rates of Professional Satisfaction and Related Constructs

Category and item	Percentage
Satisfaction, stress, and repeated choice of profession (Responding "Agree" or "Strongly agree")	
Overall, I am satisfied with my current job	81
My job is extremely stressful	47
If I were to choose over again, I would not become a physician	12
If I were to start my career over again, I would choose a different specialty	20
Intention to leave (Responding "Likely" or "Definitely")	
What is the likelihood that you will leave your current practice within TWO YEARS?	13
What is the likelihood that you will end your career as a physician (by retiring or switching to another career) within TWO YEARS?	9
Burnout (Choosing each response)	
I enjoy my work. I have no symptoms of burnout.	20
Occasionally I am under stress, and I don't always have as much energy as I once did, but I don't feel burned out.	54
I am definitely burning out and have one or more symptoms of burnout, such as physical and emotional exhaustion.	19
The symptoms of burnout that I'm experiencing won't go away. I think about frustrations at work a lot.	6
I feel completely burned out and often wonder if I can go on. I am at the point where I may need some changes or may need to seek some sort of help.	2

CHAPTER SIX

Quality of Care

Overview of Findings

In this report, we define "quality" expansively: Any activity that improves patients' chances of having good health outcomes, avoiding harm, or having good experiences with the health care system is counted as improving the quality of care. "Quality care" thus occurs when a patient gets the services that he or she needs, without unnecessary risk, in a humane and respectful manner. Drawing distinctions between specific dimensions of quality (e.g., technical quality, safety, and patient experience) is beyond the scope of this report.

Using this expansive definition of quality, we found that, when physicians perceived themselves as providing high-quality care, they were more satisfied. Conversely, obstacles to providing high-quality care were reported as major sources of professional dissatisfaction. These obstacles could originate within the practice (e.g., practice leadership that is unsupportive of quality improvement ideas) or be imposed by payers (e.g., payers that refused to cover necessary medical services).

Quantitative survey findings were generally concordant with interviewees' accounts. Physicians' self-reported ability to deliver high-quality care was statistically significantly associated with overall professional satisfaction. Receiving useful quality performance data and practice leaders' responsiveness to physicians' quality improvement suggestions were also predictors of greater professional satisfaction.

These findings suggest that, when physician dissatisfaction is attributable to perceptions of quality problems, such dissatisfaction could be viewed as a "canary in the coal mine" for health care quality—assuming that physicians are correct in their perceptions. Interventions that address physicians' quality concerns, simultaneously improving both the quality of care patients receive and physician professional satisfaction, seem likely to be attractive to multiple stakeholders. Conversely, practices in which physicians report low professional satisfaction may warrant a closer look, with the first priority being to determine whether quality problems are responsible for physician dissatisfaction.

Qualitative Findings

Providing High-Quality Care Is Inherently Satisfying

Physicians commonly reported that a great source of satisfaction for them in their work was being able to provide what they felt was high-quality care for their patients—indeed, that this was central to their desire to practice medicine. This was expressed concisely by one physician when asked for the most important factors determining professional satisfaction:

> If the patient came in, … they're not feeling good. If [I] can say anything to them to make them feel better, I feel like I did my job.
>
> —primary care physician

Being able to provide high-quality care was commonly equated with having sufficient time with patients. For example, one physician described her reasons for joining her current practice:

> [I joined this practice] because it is putting the doctor-patient relationship back at the forefront of what's important in medicine. I mean, there's a lot more to taking care of patients than just knowing which pill to give them. I mean, the whole healing art, it isn't just biochemistry. This organization allows you time to get to know your patients and also to dig deep, take care of all the details, which are important, and do a good job of it without having to work 16, 18 hours a day doing it.
>
> —primary care physician

Good relationships with patients were also important to physicians' conceptions of high-quality care, and some physicians in leadership roles explained how they had organized their practices to facilitate these relationships:

> I think one of the most rewarding things in my practice career has been the close associations you make with your patients, and in a smaller group setting you're able to spend a little bit more time with patients and get to know them. You're not a number. They know who you are, you know who they are, you know about their families, and I think that's probably … the most rewarding thing I've had out of my career.
>
> —obstetrician/gynecologist

> There's something so satisfying or something so proud about this [being] my business right here. … We're doing 100 percent of what we believe in. … I think everyone here believes, myself included, that we really do provide superior care to our patients, because it is much more individualized. [Patients] have a lot more contacts specifically with the doc, and we have a lot more continuity … and that's why we went into medicine. … It's a lot of responsibility on your shoulders and … to not be satisfied would be the worst possible [outcome]. … You've got to feel proud of what you're doing at the end of the day.
>
> —primary care physician

Perceived Barriers to Providing High-Quality Patient Care

Physicians reported dissatisfaction when there were barriers to providing high-quality care, especially when practice leadership did not support their ideas for quality improvement. As the following physician explained, pushback from practice leadership regarding steps to improve quality could be a source of frustration:

When I've been critical, I've had some pushback from [practice leadership] lately. ... For instance, we have x-ray at our clinic, and those x-rays do get read by a radiologist. But the reporting hasn't always been timely. ... So my medical assistant and I devised a system of tracking those reports to make sure that we got the reports within 24 hours, so that things weren't missed, in a timely way. ... [And] in terms of phone communication, I've asked that people who want phone calls get triaged through the medical assistant or the nurse, which happens for me. But I've gotten comments, at least in my review anyway, that people feel like I think I'm special, or that my practice is kind of special and not really fitting into the general mold of [our practice] because of that. You know, because I ask for special things. And I think those are actually things that would help the whole practice. But, for whatever reason, they've elected not to take those up. ... I actually had some pushback about having my medical assistant share an office with me, so we could coordinate and talk about things, as opposed to having the medical assistant too far away to really talk to. And it just helped me around the practice to put her in there. But it took months to actually have that happen, and [only after] some pushback.

—primary care physician

Quality problems stemming from time pressure were also a common source of dissatisfaction. The following physician explained how such problems led her to leave her previous practice:

The unrelenting pace of patient care, especially in the setting that I was in, where 70 percent of our clinic visits were [language] interpreted, ... with 15- and 20-minute visits for people who avoid seeking health care until they have serious problems, not only led to innumerable long hours, but also was an error waiting to happen. You know, there isn't time to ask all the questions that need to be asked, to do all the informed consent that needs to be done. There just isn't the time. And you do your best every single day, but you see things, you see near misses that you can do nothing about, because the system has no more capacity to reach further, and the system has no more time to help those people. So [I left the practice], after years and years of that frustration and the risk, knowing that your license could be in jeopardy at any point, even though you're trying 120 percent to do the best by everybody, because you can't catch everything at that pace.

—primary care physician

Physicians also commonly expressed dissatisfaction when they perceived payers as hindering the quality of care they provided, either due to noncoverage of necessary services or preauthorization requirements:

Well, the problem is: Who is deciding [what is medically necessary]? Somebody who's not seeing a patient. ... I had a patient today [who] was qualified for the MRI, ... but his insurance denied him because he's claustrophobic. [They] denied him the one lorazepam pill. Yeah. One pill. [They] said, "No, we're not going to pay for anything for his sedation." So then you're throwing the baby out with the bathwater, because ... if he can't stay still and you get a junky test and you get a junky answer, and then you're left with more questions than answers, well, then it doesn't help anybody. And that's what we're dealing with.

—radiologist

One physician described how these frustrations can affect the physician-patient relationship and how such frustrations can multiply:

> I think there is a lot more interference, not so much from the government, [but] from insurance companies. … [It's] extremely frustrating. [A patient has] wrenched their back taking a deck out of the lake and they've got pain radiating down into the foot and they can hardly hobble across the room and they've got positive neurologic signs, et cetera, lumbar radiculopathy, and they need an MRI. And then … it's denied. Here's a piece of paper. You've got to call this physician. You call them. You get one number, you wait and wait and wait and wait, and it's increasing encroachment on the patient-physician relationship, second guessing the things that we order. … I deal with a lot more angry patient population now because of that. It snowballs, so they don't get the medications that they need. They don't get the prior authorizations for the tests they need, the durable medical equipment, and when they don't get that, they get angry, and so we're getting a stream of patients coming in at the front desk and yelling out there because all of sudden their co-pays are going up; they're being denied medications; they're being denied medical care in much the same way that we're being denied our autonomy in ordering those things, and so there's increasing frustration on both ends, on the physicians and the patients.
>
> —primary care physician

Quantitative Findings

Among physicians responding to our survey, approximately one-half reported having practice leadership that was responsive to quality improvement suggestions, and approximately one-half received useful quality reports. Only one in seven reported feeling helpless when receiving a quality report, and three in four reported that they could provide high-quality care to all of their patients. One in seven felt overwhelmed by patients' needs. See Table 6.1.

Table 6.1
Responses to Survey Questions About Quality of Care

Item	Percentage
Responding "Agree" or "Strongly agree" to the following:	
When I suggest an idea for improving quality, this practice actually tries out the idea	51
I receive useful information about the quality of care I deliver	50
When I receive a new report about the quality of care, it just makes me feel helpless	14
It is possible to provide high quality care to all my patients	76
Formularies or prescription limits restrict the quality of care I provide	43
I am overwhelmed by the needs of my patients	15
Reporting receiving quality reports	
Quality of preventive care—own patients	53
Quality of preventive care—entire practice	45
Quality of care delivered to patients with specific conditions or who have undergone specific procedures—own patients	53
Quality of care delivered to patients with specific conditions or who have undergone specific procedures—entire practice	58

Relationships between these dimensions of quality and overall professional satisfaction generally agreed with qualitative findings. When physicians rated their practices as being more conducive to high-quality care, overall professional satisfaction was greater. Physicians who reported being overwhelmed by the needs of their patients were the least likely to report overall professional satisfaction. See Figure 6.1.

Figure 6.1
Adjusted Associations Between Physicians' Perceptions of the Quality of Care and Overall Professional Satisfaction

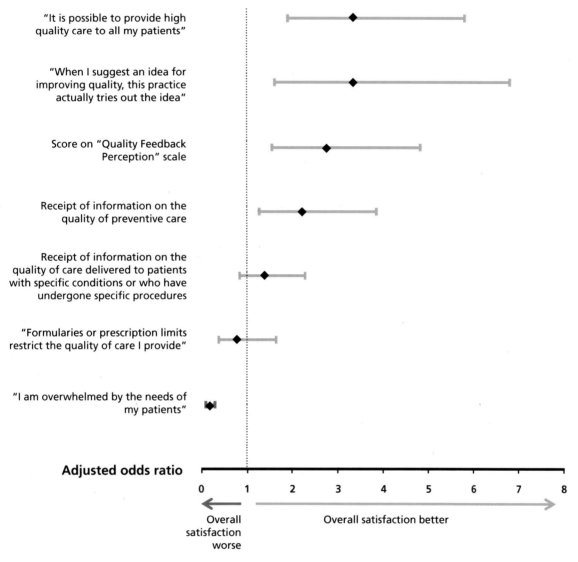

NOTES: Each estimate represents the effect of agreeing or strongly agreeing with the corresponding statement, having received individual or practice-level quality information, or a one-point increase in the corresponding continuous score (for quality feedback perceptions). Odds ratios are adjusted for practice size, specialty, and ownership, as well as for individual response tendency. 95-percent confidence intervals account for clustering of observations within practices. Statistically significant associations are highlighted by the use of colored confidence intervals: red for factors associated with worse satisfaction and green for factors associated with better satisfaction.
RAND *RR439-6.1*

Comparison Between Current Findings and Previously Published Research

Quantitative findings from the current study are similar to those from the Physician Worklife Study, which, in the 1990s, indicated that greater perceived ability to deliver high-quality patient care was associated with greater physician professional satisfaction (Linzer et al., 2000). This finding was also reported in older studies conducted among academic and clinical faculty at one academic medical center (Linn, Brook, et al., 1985; Linn, Yager, et al., 1985). We did not find previously published research investigating the relationships between physicians' receipt of quality reports and professional satisfaction.

CHAPTER SEVEN

Electronic Health Records

Overview of Findings

We found that EHRs had important effects on physician professional satisfaction, both positive and negative. In the practices we studied, physicians approved of EHRs in concept, describing better ability to remotely access patient information and improvements in quality of care. Physicians, practice leaders, and other staff also noted the potential of EHRs to further improve both patient care and professional satisfaction in the future, as EHR technology—especially user interfaces and health information exchange—improves.

However, for many physicians, the current state of EHR technology appeared to significantly worsen professional satisfaction in multiple ways. Poor EHR usability, time-consuming data entry, interference with face-to-face patient care, inefficient and less fulfilling work content, inability to exchange health information between EHR products, and degradation of clinical documentation were prominent sources of professional dissatisfaction. Some of these problems were more prominent among senior physicians and those lacking scribes, transcriptionists, and other staff to support data entry or manage information flow. Other problems, including but not limited to frustrations with receiving template-generated notes (i.e., degradation of clinical documentation), were described by physicians across the full range of specialties and practice models. In addition, EHRs have been more expensive than anticipated for some practices, threatening practice financial sustainability.

Quantitative findings from the physician survey generally were concordant with the qualitative findings; satisfaction with EHRs was an independent predictor of physicians' overall professional satisfaction. In addition, having more EHR functions, such as reminders, alerts, and messaging capabilities (a potential marker of system complexity), was associated with lower professional satisfaction.

Some practices reported taking steps to address the causes of physician dissatisfaction with EHRs. These steps were, most commonly, to allow multiple modes of data entry (including scribes and dictation with human transcriptionists) and to employ other staff members (e.g., flow managers) to help physicians focus their interactions with EHRs on activities truly requiring a physician's training.

Qualitative Findings

Among the 30 practices participating in this study, 28 were using an EHR at the time of our visits, and interviewees in these sites collectively reported their experiences with 14 different

EHR products. Below, we present the most common themes describing EHRs' effects on professional satisfaction, starting with the positive and proceeding to the negative.

Improved Professional Satisfaction: EHRs Facilitate Better Access to Patient Data

Physicians in multiple specialties and practice models noted that their EHRs improved their abilities to access patient data, both in health care settings and at home. They described this better access as improving patient care and professional satisfaction:

> There are certain efficiencies that one gains as a result of [EHRs], and universal accessibility is wonderful, particularly if you're on call at night and get called from an [emergency room] in Topeka and need to share information and even fax them something right away, it's real helpful. Those are features that are wonderful, and patients now expect it.
>
> —cardiologist

> When the system's working well, I can get to information quickly and old notes quickly. … I do like that, and I like the immediacy of having the note right there and not waiting three or four days [asking], "When is my dictation coming?" I can route it and I can send it to somebody quickly. I can print it out right away and then get it to the nursing home.
>
> —primary care physician

> You have to go way back, but yes, it was paper for a while. We had charts. We shuttled charts around in between the offices. There's no way in the world we'd go back to that. It seems barbaric now, but you would always get misplaced charts and things like that. Now, three of us in three different buildings can look at the chart at the same time. … It really is much, much better. I mean, there's no way I would go back to the old paper stuff.
>
> —primary care physician

Several physicians also noted the lifestyle advantages of accessing patient information from home.

> [Paperwork] has gotten tremendously better since we developed our electronic medical record three years ago. You can pretty much be out of here by five. Or what I will do is I will go home, have dinner, and then pull out my laptop, and that's the great thing about the electronic medical record, I can finish things that evening at my leisure.
>
> —obstetrician/gynecologist

Improved Professional Satisfaction: EHRs Improve Some Aspects of Quality of Care

Physicians and administrators in some practices described how EHRs improved their ability to provide guideline-based care and track patients' markers of disease control over time. These advantages were predominantly noted in primary care practices.

> I think [the EHR is] fantastic. … A real EHR, one that actually gives you things in fields that are usable and useful, makes all the difference. I can click a button and I can see the blood pressures over time. I'm not like thumbing through pages to say, "What was your

last blood pressure?" "Oh, and what was the one before that?" and then try to think about them. I click a button and [the EHR] graphs them for me. I can see trends. I can see what's been happening. It is incredible in facilitating communication. I mean, we have a huge practice, … and we work together as a team. How would you do that on paper?

—primary care physician

One of the quality criteria has historically been, for the diabetic, how often are they getting their hemoglobin A1C. It's a great measure, but now that we have the electronic medical record and we can see the discrete data, we can not only track, "Did the patient get it within the appropriate clinical parameter?" but we can also see where they are in the results and then track that over time. So as a patient comes to us, as a new patient, and diabetic, we are able to improve their result and improve their health just through our own medical management and then see that in the laboratory results.

—manager of a primary care practice

Improved Professional Satisfaction: Better Communication with Patients and Between Providers

Interviewees described enhanced communication through the medical record itself (e.g., by facilitating access to other providers' notes and eliminating illegible handwriting) and through EHR-based messaging applications (e.g., patient portals). Improvements in between-provider communication were most commonly noted in larger practices, where all providers were on the same EHR.

I think, if used correctly, [the EHR] definitely improves communication and helps in terms of patient care overall, with tracking what's going on with the patient. I think it's helped with patient-to-physician communication. I have a younger patient population but they love the email and, quite honestly, I have some 70- and 80-year-old patients who love the email features, who email me as well.

—primary care physician

Additionally there's a very, very sophisticated electronic medical system, with [hundreds of] docs. I'm able to look at anybody's note, anytime, on any patient that I'm interested in or that has seen me for something. I think it just erases a lot of potential for medical errors and so forth because everything is clearly documented, [and] there's not handwriting issues and so forth.

—orthopedic surgeon

Worsened Professional Satisfaction: Time-Consuming Data Entry

The majority of physicians who interacted with EHRs directly (i.e., without using a scribe or other assistant) described cumbersome, time-consuming data entry. For many physicians, voice recognition programs were not accurate enough to improve on typing. Although more-senior physicians, who tended to describe their typing skills as relatively weak, articulated these concerns most clearly, data entry was difficult for many younger physicians as well.

Physicians who used template-based notes or who used scribes were less likely to express these concerns. In the practices we visited, scribes were limited to surgeons; no other types of physicians used scribes or other staff to generate EHR notes.

One senior physician who had previously used a human transcriptionist described significant increases in the time required to generate patient notes after EHR installation:

I do not type, and I don't like [the template-based note program] at all. I don't like copying and pasting. To me, it just seems like an abomination. I'm kind of old school that way, so I chose the Dragon method of dictating so that I can put templates in [the EHR] and then dictate like I used to, and so a nice note comes out instead of a nine-page progress note under [template-based note program]. That has its own problems in that Dragon is not fully developed. It's not entirely teachable, so I spend a lot of time selecting and teaching, and there are certain [words] that I must have selected and taught [the EHR] or Dragon how to say it 50 or 60 times, and it still won't get it right and it will print things in there later that just are astonishing. … And, unfortunately, there's a lag period behind your dictation, so you can't really watch what you're dictating because then you get discombobulated, and you have to also dictate all the syntax and all the commas and everything else, so then the only other option is, after dictation, to go through the whole note and … then correcting everything and typing. Or trying to retrain just makes the dictation in the [the EHR] system very burdensome and very long, so that's mostly how it's cut back on my productivity and my time.

Interviewer: "Relative to dictating prior to [the EHR] and the Dragon system, how much more time does it take you to dictate a typical note?"

At least twice as long. … Now in the nursing home, it takes much longer, because I have to take this whole system there, log out, log in, log into their system and go through all those things just to get in, and then with each on- and off-premises charge, there are several clicks and selections to take, and if the computer is over there—if the signals are not good, it can be very, very slow. It can take me a half an hour to set up. [Before the EHR was installed,] I saw a patient in the nursing home, and then I would dictate right away using a handheld Dictaphone, and I could do the dictation in five minutes. Now it takes me at least 15 to dictate just the dictation portion of a nursing home patient. … This last weekend I worked five hours, and that was six nursing home patients it took me five hours to see. [Before the EHR], I could have seen six patients in two hours with everything—driving out there, dictation, and coming back. … It's been stressful. I think it's, the overall effect, has been to add more stress.

—primary care physician

All of the [EHRs] that I've seen have actually been very time-consuming for physicians. Physicians have to order everything themselves, which is time-consuming, and do all the data entry themselves, which is time consuming. [EHRs] at this point in the development are not time savers for physicians. They're big time sinks. Everyone agrees, everyone I talk to in every practice.

—primary care physician

Another described data entry spilling into his home life and commented on the accuracy of transcription software:

> Every screen's got 50 different things, you know, that are changing. It slows me down. So, I do a lot of my charting at night. … But, the problem is I'm spending more hours doing it than I would have before. We have Dragon, which you have to be careful of, because I just [dictated] a "Patient's prostate is bothering him" and it turned out "Patient's prostitute is bothering him." You really have to read that carefully, because I can end up going to court with that stuff.
>
> —primary care physician

Some physicians also noted that data entry had slowed work for other key members of their teams:

> The first place we started seeing [an EHR], if you will, was in operating rooms [during] the perioperative time, … where the nurse would be recording. She used to fill out a form by hand. Now it's in the computer, and everybody was like "Oh my gosh, it's taking three times as long to populate all the fields that you have to populate." … The joke early on, like on an appendix or a gallbladder or something that went really fast and easy, is: "We're done, and the nurse is over there still trying to get in the pre-op data." She has now spent 90 percent of her time at a screen, having to enter data that takes her away from circulating.
>
> —general surgeon

Worsened Professional Satisfaction: User Interfaces That Do Not Match Clinical Workflow
Beyond data entry, physicians and their colleagues described EHR user interfaces that, in important ways, hampered rather than facilitated their clinical workflow. Nonintuitive order entry was particularly problematic:

> For me, the most frustrating part is the extra time it takes. So if you have ten patients to round on, rounding on them isn't hard; it's all the order entry. … Like the other day, I discharged a patient, and I went through every step, at least I thought I did. I did everything I thought I was supposed to do, and about an hour later, I got a call from the nurse saying, "I can't discharge the patient. It won't let me finish my part." It turns out there was one button that I missed clicking, so she and I were on the phone, both on the computer looking at this patient's chart, trying to figure out why it wouldn't work. And it's just so time-consuming.
>
> —pediatrician

The cognitive load of using complex menus, pointing, and clicking was difficult for some physicians, especially while attempting to interact with patients:

> It's hard to find certain items in the computer system. [The physicians] have to click-click-click-click. They count their clicks. … It's not laid out how their workflow is, and I think it's just sometimes when you're in [the EHR] you go from page to page to page and then you forget where you started. And so you kind of get lost in the route. It's hard adjusting

to, you know, sitting in a room with a patient and having to put things in a screen while still engaging the patient.

—manager of primary care practice

Others recounted clinically important deficits in functionality and shared that software changes to address these deficits have been slow, even for some expert users:

Our particular [EHR] is buggy. There's no great way for me—say, you're my patient—I can't get your results back to you with a letter that explains what I'm thinking about, necessarily. It's like, come on, why can't we do that, you know? … I'm a diabetes educator, and I can't electronically send prescriptions for test strips and syringes and pen needles … you know, paper and pencil of my medical trade. That's what I work in, and so that's just silly. There's no reason why the drug database that we use can't do that, and sometimes the fixes are really slow in coming. … I'd been sending tickets in for months and years now: "Can we do this? Can we do this?" "Nope, sorry, you can't." … And I'm the "superuser" here. I'm the person who knows supposedly the most about this machine, and I have a lot of questions, and I wonder, if I can't do it, someone like [physician colleague], who's, like, opposed to it, who thinks it's too many clicks and too complicated and gets in the way of her relationship with her patient, what is she doing with it, you know?

—nurse practitioner

Worsened Professional Satisfaction: Interference with Face-to-Face Care

Multiple physicians who entered their notes via keyboard described their EHRs as interfering with face-to-face patient care. Many of these physicians blamed themselves for lacking the ability to type without compromising the level of attention they could devote to patients. These physicians faced a difficult trade-off: divide attention between the patient and the computer, or defer data entry until after leaving the patient, lengthening overall work hours:

[The EHR has] impacted my life incredibly, because I am not facile enough with a keyboard to be able to talk to somebody and type at the same time, and it's too important for me to be able to communicate with my patients and see how they're reacting to [what I'm saying]. I mean, you know, I can't tell how depressed they are while I'm doing this and looking at a computer screen and they're sitting behind me. So I don't do my notes while I'm in the room, although that's the goal—that the physicians are supposed to be able to do their notes as they're talking to the patient. I'm sure people who are more facile with this technology probably can do that. I can't, so I finish my day and then I have several hours' worth of typing ahead of me, which is a real drag.

—primary care physician

I find [the EHR] inefficient in that I used to write the note [on paper] while I was in the room with the patient, and I would say, "I'm going to write while I'm here, is that okay with you?" And people will generally appreciate that. I can't type and not look at the screen, just not a thing I can do. And I don't like the idea of having technology there, same reason I don't have it at my dinner table. And so, in that regard, it makes me less efficient, because I can't just leave the room and have things already written and a plan already in my mind and write three sentences and be finished with the note. Instead, I interact with the patient, touch the patient, look at the patient in the eyes and then I come out of the room and interact with the computer.

—hospitalist

Worsened Professional Satisfaction: Insufficient Health Information Exchange

Physicians in multiple specialties and a range of practice settings described frustration when health information was not exchanged between EHRs. Even when practices invested in EHRs, faxes were a common mode of communicating patient information between care settings:

We still get things faxed, and so we get the paper. Then the paper we have to … scan it into the system. So it hasn't really saved us completely from paper. I've been in the system now two years, about, and still we have papers. We still have to scan, every day we have to do this. And plus the systems that you work with, not all of them talk to each other, as you know. … So also when the labs come, you know we have only one lab now that talks to us. So if people do labs different places then it comes in the form of [a] fax. … And also, we don't have, yet, radiologist systems that talk to us. So it's always again, it's a fax, same thing scanned in.

—primary care physician

One physician wondered why interoperability was not a regulatory requirement:

The hospitals have a different EHR, and they don't communicate, which was the big problem, I think, in [health reform—] … it did not mandate [interoperable] electronic records. The best thing they should have done was to pick a couple organizations and [say]: "You're going to [create] electronic medical records, and you need to all communicate easily." That way we can get stuff from the hospital and everything else. … That's, I think, the big problem: Everyone's going to electronic medical records, [but] there's not an easy way for everything to communicate. And I think that was kind of the purpose behind it, that people could have their history and it'd be portable and they could go from place to place and everyone would be able to see what's been done and not duplicate it and be up to date on what was going on with that patient.

—general surgeon

In some cases, having multiple EHRs and other computer systems within a given practice also limited information flow, frustrating physicians:

The biggest limitations come from our lack of good interfaces and the fact that the hospital has way too many different computer systems. So for instance, our scheduling system, which is from 1994—oh, my God, makes me want to cry—doesn't interface perfectly with [our EHR]. And so when a patient cancels [an appointment], you can't always tell they've canceled on your [EHR] schedule. We order everything electronically, and then our secretaries print it out and transfer it to another system. So there are operational problems that I think are not related to the system itself being inadequate, but our [information technology] infrastructure at the hospital [is also] inadequate. … For instance, all the labs we order come back to [our EHR], all the radiology we order comes back to [our EHR]. The colonoscopies do not, because that will be another system. Because, of course, [gastroenterology] is functioning in their own little silo, and we'd need to build another interface to our system.

—primary care physician

Worsened Professional Satisfaction: Information Overload

Some EHR products feature automatic email alerts to physicians. For primary care physicians in particular, this has created a sense of information overload—the unceasing volume of messages reaching them has expanded beyond the number that they believe they can handle diligently:

I think the most important challenge [with the EHR] is physician satisfaction. Since we switched to the EMR, you know, everything comes in that box. It's like just ding, ding, ding, ding. When you go away for a week and you come back, there is just so much [email] volume to go through, and that's a big dissatisfier with physicians. ... The culprit is the [EHR], the computer. ... Everything that happens to the patient is there; they keep sending [it]. Every podiatry visit, every nutritionist visit, every specialist visit, whatever they did, keeps coming, and it's in multiple places. ... Faxes come, they send you an ER report, the x-ray, and the CAT scan. And the moment you click it, you own it. And you make sure there's nothing wrong there, ... because if you missed it, you're in trouble, okay? And this goes on every day. So the volume of the stuff you have to go through is out of control. ... My point is there's an overload of information which is not necessary, ... if you go and see the podiatrist, nutritionist, their notes will be in the [EHR], it's not going anywhere. It's there. But why do you have to send it to me [via EHR-generated email as well]? ... By end of the day, if I clear my desk, [and] I go home, there'll be another 10, 15 labs or something sitting [in my inbox]. And then by morning it becomes 30. [If] you don't clear 30 today, tomorrow it'll be 60. That's how it multiplies. ... So you're like, run, run, run, and the older you get, how fast can you run? Mentally, I mean, not physically. So that's what happens. So it's had its own, you know, stress. That's one of the reasons why you saw that the satisfaction [decreased].

—primary care physician

Worsened Professional Satisfaction: Mismatch Between Meaningful-Use Criteria and Clinical Practice

Both primary care and subspecialist physicians noted a mismatch between meaningful-use criteria and what they considered to be the most important elements of patient care.[1] Some physicians who did not provide primary care reported that meaningful-use criteria seemed to be more appropriate to primary care practice. However, primary care physicians also reported that the documentation burden of satisfying meaningful-use criteria detracted from patient care:

I think [the EHR] was created to get us a gold star for "meaningful use" but not to make it easy for a physician [with] on boots on the ground to use it. ... They really aren't really hitting their user group very well. I think, for me, one of the big frustrations is there are so

---

[1] *Meaningful-use criteria* refer to the requirements for EHR use that physicians must satisfy to receive payments under the EHR incentive program of the American Recovery and Reinvestment Act of 2009.

many things that I need to put in there now. ... I have to make sure all the i's are dotted and the t's are crossed, because we want to make sure we're hitting on all of our measures. ... And so it requires that probably half the time that I'm charting, I'm dotting those i's and crossing those t's and making sure that I work the chart, which is not taking care of patients. ... I'd rather spend that time face to face. ... So I think what we've created is almost a monster, when really what we were shooting for was good patient care. And that's unfortunate.

—primary care physician

Worsened Professional Satisfaction: EHRs Threaten Practice Finances

Some physicians, especially those who owned or who were partners in their practices, reported that investing in EHRs exposed their practices to significant financial risks. In particular, the costs of switching EHRs—which could become necessary due to factors beyond a practice's control—were of high concern:

The downside is cost. I mean, the cost is tremendous. And you know there are competing companies out there, but that doesn't necessarily mean that they have a better product. And if you switch to a competing company, you just have to start from scratch. And the cost for what they offer is just astronomical. And there's no way to put a price tag on it. I mean, you can compare cars and figure out what price you want to pay for this car versus that car, even if they're different models, but you can't do that with EHRs. ... And we have been involved with [EHR vendor] since the beginning of our EHR, and [EHR vendor] has been going through some changes at a corporate level as well. So you're always worried, what's going to happen with [EHR vendor]? Are they going to get bought out by somebody else? Are they going to cease to exist? Or are they going to continue to service their product? It's very worrisome.

—primary care physician

Other physicians in practice management positions expressed concern about the ongoing costs of maintaining their EHRs. These upkeep costs were a particularly pressing problem in smaller practices that could not afford dedicated information technology personnel, as the following practice owner described:

[The EHR] is not just a one-time investment. It is a hugely expensive, ongoing, every freaking day investment. So over the years, I have ... spent probably three quarters of a million dollars since [adopting our] electronic medical record, because every year, you pay 20 percent of the value of it. And there's sometimes between 8 and 15,000 dollars a year in support fees. There's new computers. I think we have 16 computers, and every year we probably have to replace at least three to five of them. The printers. The IT support to come get everything connected. When we moved [to our new office], we bought a new server. A year later, with "meaningful use," my vendor said "Guess what? Your server doesn't work with that. Now you have to buy another 12,000 dollar server." ... Because we're small, we don't really have an IT person. [The IT person], scarily, is me, and I'm like the least qualified person in the room to be the IT person. And then if you want to get somebody who is that qualified IT person, you're looking at several thousand dollars a month. Well, a practice this size can't really justify somebody that's 2,000 dollars a month for IT support.

—primary care physician

Worsened Professional Satisfaction: EHRs Require Physicians to Perform Lower-Skilled Work

Physicians who did not use scribes reported that their EHRs required them to perform tasks below their level of training, decreasing their efficiency:

I'm not a clerk. At least, I don't think I am. I'm more efficient calling [a clerk] into the room and saying, "Okay, set up Mrs. Jones for tests A, B, C, D and F," and you go do it. I don't know how long it takes you, but what I do know is that I'm done, I'm moving on, as opposed to when [I enter the order myself]: A click, B click, C click, D click. Oh, I need to give a reason for D, open up the box, click, click, click, click, okay, close the box, and verify, and quantify, oh, and commit, so that we get "meaningful use" out of my interaction. That takes time. Am I more efficient than the world at large? Yes. But am I a clerk? No. So, everything is just a couple of clicks, but if you followed me around and looked at how many "couple of clicks" tasks I do, it takes time. And I could do all that, but then there's a personal value decision. I prefer to look at you [the patient] when I'm talking to you, [rather] than look at the computer screen and glance at you sideways. So, I'm either a dinosaur, or a slow adopter, or there's something wrong with our EHR efficiency concept.

—cardiologist

In addition to frustration with the inefficiency of having physicians perform tasks that others could perform, some physicians reported a more basic emotional response:

What's really happened is since going on [the EHR] is that I've really taken on the responsibility of transcription as well as billing, in addition to the other things. … It's given me more mundane clerk-like duties to do. The derogatory term, I guess, in residency, was "scutwork." And that's what [the EHR] has done.

—primary care physician

Worsened Professional Satisfaction: Template-Based Notes Degrade the Quality of Clinical Documentation

While some physicians described using templates (or "macros") to ease the writing of clinical notes (i.e., to overcome data entry problems), many described misuse of template-based notes as a significant threat to both clinical quality and professional satisfaction. Such notes were described as complicating the task of retrieving useful clinical information. This problem was reported by physicians in all specialties and practice models included in the study:

We've been in the [EHR] system for what must be almost three years now. It's hard to believe it's been that long. And how do we like it? … As with all electronic medical records, I greatly dislike the document that's produced. We live in a world now where almost every provider, or at least I would say the majority of the providers around here, seem to have electronic systems, none of which are particularly easy to interpret. And it is a source of general,

I think, dissatisfaction among the physicians that we have been forced to abandon [a way of documentation] that was always very effective and very succinct. And the days of being able to dictate in a meaningful fashion, in the form of a letter or a concise document to send to a primary care doctor, are gone, and that's lamentable, because that has been a step down in quality. These new documents are unreadable because you've got to skim through them really quickly and say, "Where's the meat here?"

—cardiologist

I don't think anybody's found that "better [documentation]" means quicker unless [doctors are] just using some completely macro note [in which] you just pull things in and don't have any additional input. ... I mean, just a lot of the crap [is] in there when I get [notes from] consultants. Ninety-five percent of what I get back is just BS, pulled in from a chart somewhere with no thought involved.

—primary care physician

In some cases, physicians reported that template-based notes introduced enough false information to cast doubt on the medical record more broadly:

So here's what's happened with the EHR. I mean I get it, I understand it, but it has been a step backwards, I think—and as big a step backwards as it is forwards. The step backwards is the problem of templated information. ... There's templated information in the review of systems. [I think:] "Really? You asked all those questions?" Not really. "Well, what percent? 80?... 70?... 60?... 30?... Did you ask *any* questions, really?"

—general surgeon

Future Effects on Professional Satisfaction: Physicians Express Optimism About EHR Development in the Long Term

Almost universally within our study sample, physicians reported support for EHRs in concept. Some physicians hoped that future developments in artificial intelligence and health information exchange would solve problems with current EHRs:

All of a sudden, you've got this incredible goliath of information that is interfering with the ability to communicate between providers what they need to be able to communicate. So it's in transition, and I know that 10 years from now or 15 or 20 years from now, I can imagine that the next level of EHR is going to be software, smart software that can scan an eight-page document and then give me a third of a page summary of important information, because there was some software engineer who's medically trained. That, to me, makes the next logical step. Then also complete interconnectivity and transfer of information across all systems, ... so that we're not constantly reloading and scanning. [But currently] we're in a very difficult, rudimentary phase of conversion to the EHR that quite honestly has, I think, been a bigger headache than advantage for physicians, and the only reason they did it was because there was some dollars assigned to it.

—general surgeon

Quantitative Findings

Our initial clinician survey, fielded to the first six practices we visited, did not include electronic health records as a major focus. However, we discovered through our qualitative interviews that, in each of the first six practices we visited, physicians and other staff described EHRs as important determinants of professional satisfaction. Therefore, we added items specifically assessing respondents' experiences with EHRs to the clinician survey and fielded this revised survey to the remaining 24 practices.

Among these 24 practices, 22 used EHRs, and we analyzed physicians' responses to survey items concerning use of EHRs within these 22 practices. We found that most physicians relied heavily on EHRs and believed they improved the quality of care. While the physicians in our sample were dissatisfied with certain aspects of their EHRs, only one in five preferred paper records to EHRs. See Table 7.1.

As shown in Figure 7.1, physician satisfaction with EHRs is associated with overall professional satisfaction. Physicians who reported that their EHRs slowed their clinical work, who preferred paper records to EHRs, who received an overwhelming number of electronic messages, or who reported that their EHRs interfered with face-to-face patient care were the least likely to report high overall professional satisfaction. There were trends toward better overall professional satisfaction when EHRs were perceived as improving the quality of care and worse professional satisfaction when EHRs were perceived requiring physicians to perform tasks that others could perform.

In our sample, there was no significant relationship between overall satisfaction and the length of time since EHR installation. In addition, physicians whose practices reported having

Table 7.1
Responses to Survey Questions About Electronic Health Records

Item	Percentage
Responding "Agree" or "Strongly agree" to the following:	
Our electronic health record improves my job satisfaction	35
In our practice, our electronic health record improves the quality of care	61
Our electronic health record requires me to perform tasks that other staff could perform	61
Using an electronic health record enhances patient-doctor communication that is not face-to-face	54
When I am providing clinical care, our electronic health record slows me down	43
Our electronic health record improves my job satisfaction	38
Using an electronic health record interferes with patient-doctor communication during face-to-face clinical care	36
I receive an overwhelming number of electronic messages in this practice	31
Based on my experience to date, I prefer using paper medical records instead of electronic records	18

NOTE: "Overall satisfaction with EHR" is the mean of the above items on their original Likert scales (with appropriate items reverse-scored to maintain consistent directional meaning).

Figure 7.1
Adjusted Associations Between Physicians' Ratings of Their EHRs and Overall Professional Satisfaction

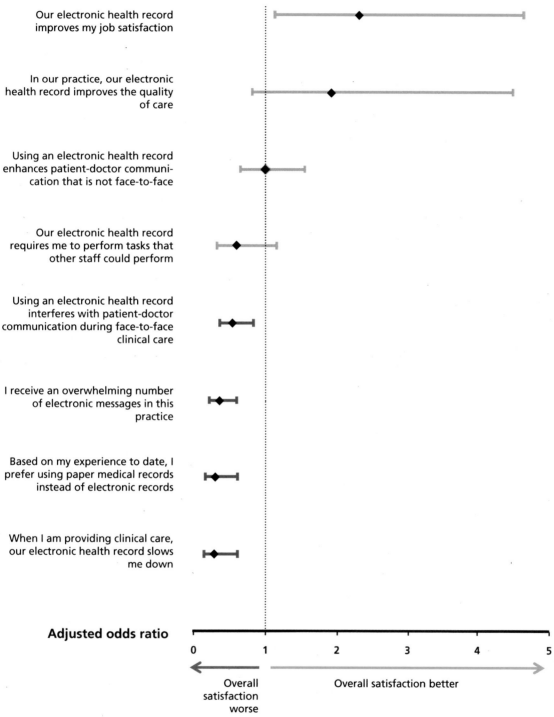

NOTES: Each estimate represents the effect of agreeing or strongly agreeing with the corresponding statement. Odds ratios are adjusted for practice size, specialty, and ownership, as well as for individual respondent seniority (number of years in practice) and response tendency. 95-percent confidence intervals account for clustering of observations within practices. Statistically significant associations are highlighted by the use of colored confidence intervals: red for factors associated with worse satisfaction and green for factors associated with better satisfaction.

RAND *RR439-7.1*

greater numbers of EHR functions (with higher numbers indicating more advanced and possibly more complex EHRs) were less likely to have high overall professional satisfaction. This finding was robust to adjustment for all confounders except practice ownership (physician ownership was collinear with having fewer EHR functions). See Figure 7.2.

Comparison Between Current Findings and Previously Published Research

Although some physicians have used EHRs for more than a decade, nationwide financial incentives to implement EHRs with certain functionalities are relatively new. As a result, literature describing how EHRs affect physician satisfaction is sparse. A 2005 survey of Florida physicians found that better satisfaction was associated with EHR and personal data assistant (e.g., PalmPilot) use, but worse satisfaction was associated with using email to communicate with their patients (Menachemi, Powers and Brooks, 2009). A survey of Massachusetts physicians conducted in 2005 found that physicians whose practices had EHRs were more likely to report dissatisfaction (Quinn et al., 2009). In a second survey of Massachusetts physicians conducted in 2007, 30 percent of physicians reported that their EHRs created new opportunities for error, but only 2 percent reported that their EHRs created more errors than they prevented (Love

Figure 7.2
Adjusted Associations Between Duration of EHR Use, EHR Feature Count, and Overall Professional Satisfaction

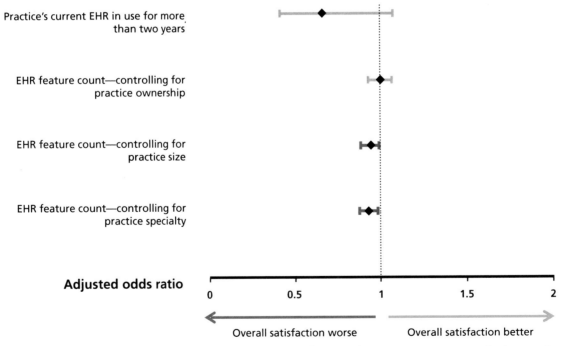

NOTES: Each estimate represents the effect of having an EHR for more than two years or a one-point increase in the number of EHR features at the practice. Odds ratios are adjusted for practice size, specialty, and ownership, as well as for individual response tendency. 95-percent confidence intervals account for clustering of observations within practices. Statistically significant associations are highlighted by the use of colored confidence intervals: red for factors associated with worse satisfaction and green for factors associated with better satisfaction.
RAND *RR439-7.2*

et al., 2012). In this 2007 survey, physician perception of new EHR-generated opportunities for error was associated with lower odds of reporting overall satisfaction with current practice.

To our knowledge, the current study is the first to investigate the relationship between EHR use, EHR ratings by physicians, and professional satisfaction across a range of geographic settings following the passage of the American Recovery and Reinvestment Act of 2009.

However, multiple prior studies that did not investigate the relationships between overall professional satisfaction and EHR use have also found the types of specific problems the physicians in the current study described: increased documentation time and interference with face-to-face patient care (El-Kareh et al., 2009; Fernandopulle and Patel, 2010), inaccurate information in template-based (or copied) notes (Hirschtick, 2006), mismatch to clinical workflow, barriers to health information exchange (Adler-Milstein, Bates and Jha, 2013; O'Malley et al., 2010), threats to overall practice finances (Adler-Milstein, Green and Bates, 2013), and a variety of usability problems (Koppel et al., 2005; Koppel, 2013; Middleton et al., 2013; Johnson, 2006; Fernandopulle and Patel, 2010). The Institute of Medicine and others have begun to outline approaches for addressing EHR usability in the context of clinical workflow (Middleton et al., 2013; Institute of Medicine, 2012; Sinsky et al., 2013; Armijo, McDonnell and Werner, 2009).

In a longitudinal study of these perceptions over a 12-month period following EHR implementation conducted among primary care physicians in 2006–2008 within a single large physician group in Massachusetts, these problems declined in prevalence (e.g., the proportion of physicians reporting that EHRs increased their documentation time fell from 78 percent to 68 percent), and perceptions of EHRs' benefits increased (El-Kareh et al., 2009). The persistence of reported EHR problems in the current study, even in practices that had implemented EHRs several years prior to our interviews, and our inability to detect a statistically significant relationship between professional satisfaction and years since EHR installation (using a two-year threshold) are not directly comparable to these earlier findings but do not appear to conflict with them.

Autonomy and Work Control

Overview of Findings

Greater physician autonomy and greater control over the pace and content of clinical work were both associated with better professional satisfaction. For some physicians, having a leadership or management role within the practice was a key way of achieving autonomy. However, practice ownership was not for everyone: Some physicians reported little taste for the business side of medicine, deriving satisfaction from employed positions that allowed them to focus more exclusively on clinical care.

In general, analyses of survey results were concordant with interviewee reports; physicians reporting greater degrees of control over their clinical work were more likely to also report high overall professional satisfaction.

Because interviewees reported that practice structure and ownership could facilitate or limit their autonomy and ability to control their work, we also investigated the relationships between practice model and overall satisfaction. Among the practice descriptors we studied within our sample, ownership model was a significant predictor of satisfaction: Physicians in physician-owned practices or partnerships were more likely to be satisfied than those in other ownership models (hospital or corporate ownership). Restricting our analyses just to practices with hospital or corporate ownership, we found that relationships between autonomy, work control, and overall satisfaction were similar to the overall sample. This finding suggests that, in hospital- or corporate-owned practices, strategies to enhance physicians' abilities to control the factors immediately affecting their day-to-day clinical work may be important to preserving or enhancing professional satisfaction within these increasingly common practice configurations.

Qualitative Findings

Ability to Choose Colleagues and Coworkers

Physicians reported greater professional satisfaction when they were able to choose their colleagues and coworkers. For example, physicians placed importance on being able to choose the allied health professionals with whom they worked. The following physician, now working in a practice that recently had been acquired by a hospital, described how having a reduced ability to decide on staffing led to frustration:

> The [former owner-physicians] don't decide on hiring, firing, or even ... placement of individuals in the clinic. ... For some of my colleagues, it's been hard for them, because they feel like they need more help, [but] they're not able to just ... say, "Hey, put another

person here." They don't have that control. So, sometimes they feel frustrated that they can't manage the support staff like they would like to. ... There was more input [into staffing decisions in the past]. Now, it's more: "Make do with what you got."

—primary care physician

For some physicians, inability to choose members of their care teams led to departure from a previous practice:

I want to be independent. I want to make decisions that are right for myself and my patients, and I don't want to go through a big bureaucracy in trying to get things done. When you're employed, you're limited to that. In fact, when I started [in another practice], I didn't ... even have a lot of choice about my immediate staff. ... When I was employed, I saw three [medical] assistants come and go [without my input]. ... So I decided it was the right time to become independent.

—primary care physician, owner of current practice

Physicians also noted the importance of being able to select the other physicians in the practice:

For a partnership, it's a 100 percent vote in our bylaws. ... I don't believe we should take a partner with a partial vote. It needs to be unanimous. That's a huge decision. Everybody should get their say in that one.

—orthopedic surgeon

Selectivity regarding physician colleagues was especially important to practice reputation and sustainability, as one physician explained:

I always think that if we get one bad provider in here, that could really mess things up ... because then the reputation goes down. People won't trust us anymore. Like, ... "They don't care, they just take your money every month." Or, "I had this horrible outcome" or "I was supposed to see the doctor for 30 minutes, but he only saw me for 10, and then he rushed me out the door." ... So if we get one doctor like that, I think that it'll be bad for everyone.

—primary care physician

Primary care physicians also valued having the ability to refer patients to colleagues of their choosing:

We tend to, as a group, be very picky about the specialists we send our patients to, and we talk internally about who we think has a better bedside manner and who we think is a more thorough specialist. ... We tend to really try to direct people to individuals [rather than institutions] because we feel pretty protective of our patients out there.

—primary care physician

Control Over Business and Managerial Decisions

Physicians varied widely in their degree of interest in the business and managerial aspects of running a practice. Some physicians described an inherent enjoyment of the business side of medicine and the independence that being business owners gave them. As one practice co-owner described:

> There's something so satisfying or something so proud about this [being] my business right here. … We're doing 100 percent of what we believe in. … There are hard decisions to be made, but you can't get mad at anyone else; you're the one who's making the decisions. There's not a memo coming down from above telling you, "By the way, you work Saturdays now"—or something along those lines. … That's why we went into medicine. … It's a lot of responsibility on your shoulders and … to not be satisfied would be the worst possible [outcome]. … You've got to feel proud of what you're doing at the end of the day.
>
> —primary care physician

Even without practice ownership, some employed physicians described enjoying the management roles that were created by leading quality improvement projects:

> You hope going into [an improvement project] that the part that you're going to do on the admin side is to help make practice management better [and] make patient care better. … I've always been kind of a leader and someone that's okay in administrative "boss-type" positions. … It also is going to give me some opportunities just to see the [management] side of health care, … so it's going to be a nice big challenge.
>
> —primary care physician

Physicians reported that authority over certain financial decisions was especially important. Key among these were capital investments deemed necessary for patient care and the ability to determine salaries for physician and staff within the practice. This physician described the autonomy for making such capital investments in a small group practice as being a source of satisfaction:

> One of the nice things about this [practice] is that … if I need a new [electrocardiogram] machine, I just buy it. I might look around to try and find the best price or something, but nobody's going to say we can't do it. It's a wonderful thing to have some control.
>
> —primary care physician

Similarly, the following administrator of a practice that had recently been acquired by a hospital described a new inability to make certain capital investments in a timely manner:

> When we were private, we'd have our own shareholders meeting, and if we wanted to buy a new ultrasound, they'd vote on it, and I'd go buy a new ultrasound. Well, now … it may take us six months to get it … so I guess [the physicians] gave up some of their control.
>
> —practice administrator

This cardiology practice leader described the importance of maintaining control over internal financial decisions, such as how physicians are compensated, even after the practice had been acquired by a larger hospital entity:

The model that we chose, which was the PSA [professional services agreement], was chosen for a couple of reasons, not the least of which was to be able to maintain our autonomy as much as possible. ... We were able to negotiate a position in which, first of all, we controlled the payments and the salaries of all of our employees and of our docs, so we were paid as a practice but we decided how that money was allocated. That's a huge thing, not to have the hospital be able to say, "You need to get rid of So-and-So and So-and-So," and you need to jettison two doctors because they are not performing. And we were able to negotiate an [internal] compensation model that was, we think, fair.

—cardiologist, practice leader

Interviewees also described a significant population of physicians who had less interest in practice management, preferring to focus on clinical activities exclusively. For such physicians, employment within a practice that did not require them to perform management activities was a source of satisfaction. As one physician explained:

Those who come to work here are mostly "Okay, I will do my job, send me a paycheck and I don't want to worry about billing, I don't worry about hiring or firing, nothing. Give me an out." So there's some different type of physician who likes to work in a large group like this. ... But doctors [are] happy because they say, "Leave me alone, I want to do my job. Pay me my salary. I don't want to hire, fire, build, nothing."

—primary care physician

In this vein, the following pediatrician reported that joining a larger practice had provided a degree of insulation from external forces and allowed a renewed focus on clinical activities:

With [larger organization] acquiring us, some changes definitely came along with that. But again, the not needing to worry about all the administrative stuff, where I get just to do medicine, you know, I like that a lot. Because we are in such a big corporation, a lot of things get absorbed that I don't have to worry about. ... There's a lot of buffering that happens with the economy and decisions made about the reimbursement and stuff with insurance companies. That mostly gets absorbed, you know, by the larger corporation, the larger group.

—pediatrician

However, several physicians with less inherent interest in business matters wanted to know basic information about practice finances. The following physician described how a desire to receive information on practice finances led to joining a smaller practice:

Even though I'm not involved in the operations from a financial standpoint, knowing all the ins and outs of the books, I still wanted to have some involvement in [financial matters] and know what's going on, and I felt like that'd be a lot easier to do in a smaller practice.

—primary care physician

Ability to Earn Desired Income

Although physicians in our study did not attach specific dollar amounts to their satisfaction, they valued having control over the amount of income they earned and being able to make their own trade-offs between incomes and hours worked:

> When I came out [of training], I felt like I was working hard, ... but I wasn't making the money that I needed for overhead. And some of those numbers came in, and I was like, "Oh my gosh, what do I do?" You work harder. ... Just turn the knobs right. I just started working even harder. And, you know, it paid off. So you start seeing the pattern: The harder I work, the more I make. And it was challenging in the beginning. ... I enjoy private practice. I like the freedom, so to speak. You know, I can look at my year and almost pick out when I'm going to take my vacation and days off if I want them. Just that flexibility. ... I really enjoy the flexibility, the freedom.
>
> —orthopedic surgeon

> I didn't really care what my guaranteed salary was going to be, starting out. ... Because my attitude was, "I'm willing to work." I work hard. I put in more than a hundred percent all the time, willing to always accommodate, and I wasn't worried about my guarantee. ... To me, it was the upside potential, and "How much control did I have over my ability to see patients?" and "Were there things that were going to get in the way?
>
> —primary care physician

Ability to Choose Hours and Schedule

In all specialties and practice models included in this study, physicians valued having control over their work hours and schedules. Physicians expressed dissatisfaction when hours and schedules were perceived as overly rigid or when physicians did not have input into certain aspects of patient scheduling. For example, the following physician reported that, despite the benefits of implementing same-day access, this change also gave her less control over her schedule, compromising the quality and efficiency of care in some cases:

> Increasingly, my practice has been shaped and modified by folks that place patients into the schedule without my foreknowledge or my ability to manage the encounter before I see them. ... This same-day access has been designed, I think, favorably for patients to feel like they can be seen quickly. But sometimes, in order to make it work, there are folks who do the appointing and the scheduling but don't actually know the patients, and so some of the nuances may not be fully appreciated. The dilemma when people are double-booked, or a very complicated patient is placed in a short time schedule, is that it makes it hard to [stay on time for the other patients on my schedule]. And sometimes I might have wished that I had known about [a specific patient] earlier so that I could create some groundwork and order some things before I actually saw [the patient].
>
> —primary care physician

Some respondents believed that the degree to which a practice was able to be responsive to physician and providers' need for flexibility in the schedule and the work hours was related to the ownership structure of the practice. The following practice administrator at a physician-owned organization reported:

> Once you come on as employed, you're sort of treated as a partner even if you're not there yet. ... They don't really put boundaries in there. ... We're small enough that it's doable, it's manageable. They are actually looking at right now changing their call schedule so that they have a set day off here ... because physicians wanted some sort of ability to schedule outside of work with some consistency. And so that was driven by what they wanted. ... I think that's basically the biggest thing that they do for physician satisfaction: They'll work on any idea that comes up our way. If [a physician] has the idea, we'll look at it. There's no "No's."
>
> —practice administrator

Importantly, physicians demonstrated willingness to embrace creative solutions to filling the changing scheduling needs of a practice given the requirements of new models of care, such as open access scheduling and extended hours:

> From a physician satisfaction perspective ... it's also big for organizations to try to embrace part-time physicians a little bit more. ... So if you're trying to do more open access and hours for patients, okay, maybe there's two part-time physicians that want to do that, but they're not going to want to work five days a week, 7 a.m. to 7 p.m. So let's share a practice or let's work together as a practice.
>
> —primary care physician

Similarly, these physicians described the importance of being able to negotiate a flexible schedule in order to engage in activities outside of the practice of medicine:

> I negotiated with [practice leader] to extend the lunch so that I could go to the gym on Mondays and then extended the day half an hour at the end, so to compensate for that. ... And that keeps me sane. Tuesday and Thursday, I have half days so I do that on my time, and Friday, I end at 3:00 and go to the gym after that. So I'm able to maintain that important piece of balance in my life.
>
> —primary care physician

> I think the autonomy is probably number one, especially for somebody like myself. I have two young kids. So my son is graduating from 5th grade. I said, "I'm not working that day." I don't have to ask. I don't have to put it on the schedule. Somebody can't say [my request for time off] was too late. And so I try to be home. I work a whole lot, but when there are special occasions I can adjust my schedule accordingly. And that part I really cherish. ... And it really all comes down to autonomy.
>
> —general surgeon

Quantitative Findings

Among physicians responding to our survey, approximately one in four reported having substantial opportunities to participate in major strategic decisions affecting the practice. One in five devoted at least 10 percent of his or her work hours to management activities, and one in ten devoted at least 20 percent of work hours to management. Respondents reported a wide range of scores on established scales reflecting autonomy and work control. See Table 8.1.

Congruent with our qualitative findings, physicians' individual ratings of their abilities to control their work were statistically significantly associated with better overall satisfaction, and there were similar trends for having opportunities to participate in strategic decisions. In addition, there was a nonsignificant trend toward better professional satisfaction as the share of physicians' work hours devoted to management increased. See Figure 8.1.

Because some interviewees reported that their practice models could facilitate or limit their autonomy and work control, we also investigated the relationships between practice model and overall satisfaction. Among the practice descriptors we studied in our sample, ownership model was the only significant predictor. Physicians in physician-owned practices or partnerships were more likely to be satisfied than those in other ownership models (hospital, corporate). This association diminished in magnitude and statistical significance after adjustment for work control and opportunities to participate in strategic decisions, suggesting that these factors are partial mediators of the effect of practice ownership on overall professional satisfaction. See Figure 8.2.

Restricting our analyses just to practices with hospital or corporate ownership, we reanalyzed the relationships between markers of autonomy and work control and professional satisfaction. As in the overall sample, we found that work control was a significant predictor of professional satisfaction, but opportunities to participate in strategic decisions were not (perhaps because physicians choosing hospital- or corporate-owned practices are less interested in the "business" aspects of medical practice). These findings suggest that strategies to enhance physicians' work control may be important to preserving or enhancing professional satisfaction within these growing ownership models. See Figure 8.3.

Comparison Between Current Findings and Previously Published Research

Findings from the current study agree with those in a number of studies finding greater professional satisfaction when physicians have greater control over their work schedules (Buchbinder

Table 8.1
Responses to Survey Questions Relevant to Autonomy and Work Control

Item	Percentage
Responding "Agree" or "To a great extent" to the following:	
"I have opportunities to participate in major strategic decisions (like partnering or merging with another practice or hospital)"	26
Physicians reporting	
10 percent or more of total work hours devoted to management activities	21
20 percent or more of total work hours devoted to management activities	9

Figure 8.1
Adjusted Associations Between Physicians' Autonomy, Work Control, and Management Activities

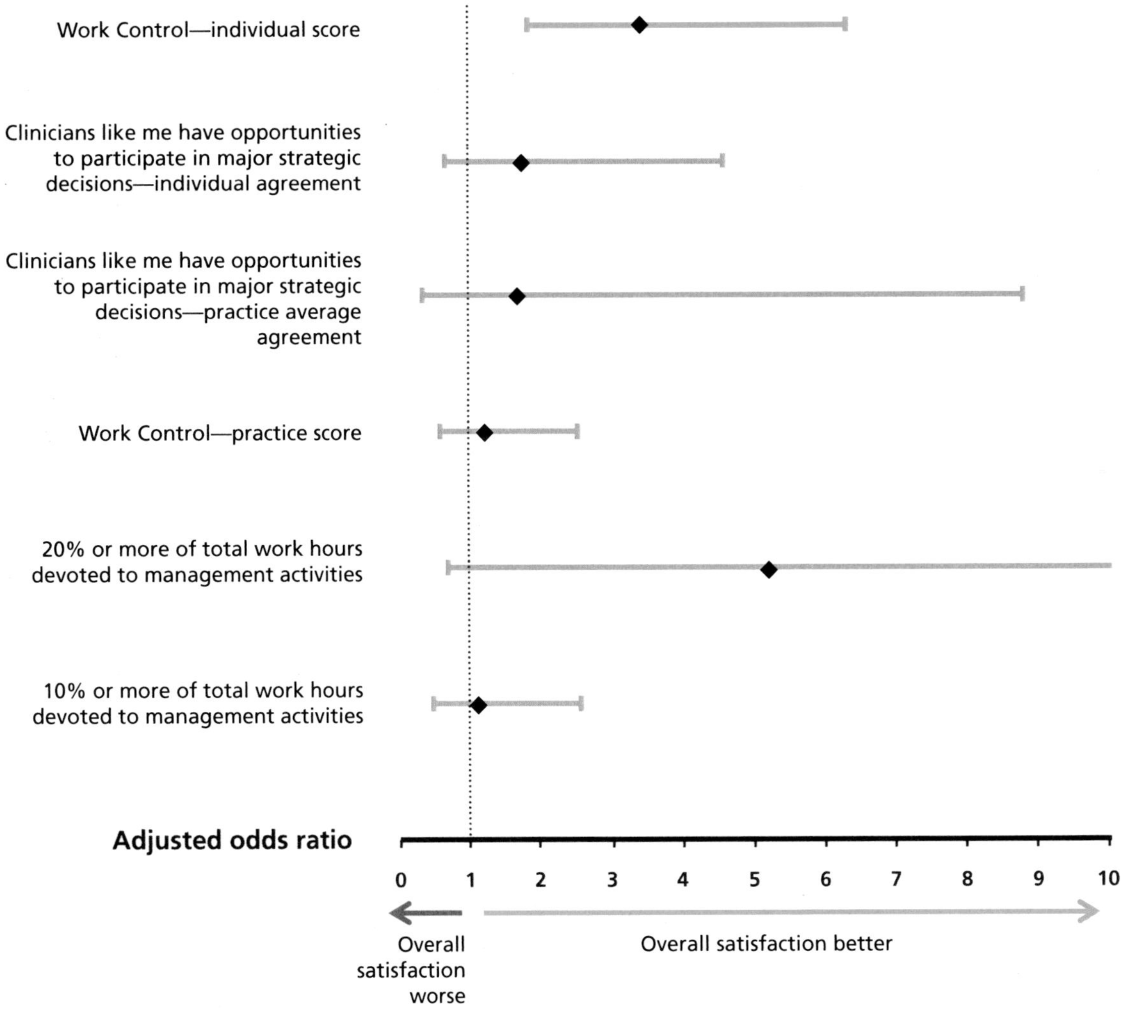

NOTES: Each estimate represents the effect of a one-point increase in the corresponding continuous score, agreeing or strongly agreeing with the corresponding statement, or devoting the corresponding share of work hours to management activities. Odds ratios are adjusted for practice size, specialty, and ownership, as well as for individual response tendency. 95-percent confidence intervals account for clustering of observations within practices. Statistically significant associations are highlighted by the use of colored confidence intervals: red for factors associated with worse satisfaction and green for factors associated with better satisfaction.
RAND RR439-8.1

et al., 2001), greater autonomy (Warren, Weitz and Kulis, 1998), control over work content (Landon, Reschovsky and Blumenthal, 2003), and other measures of work control (Linzer et al., 2002; Cydulka and Korte, 2008; Linzer et al., 2009).

The current study's quantitative findings regarding practice ownership and professional satisfaction differ from those in the most recent published analysis of Community Tracking Study/Health Tracking Physician Survey data from 2004–2005, which indicated no statistically significant difference in satisfaction between physicians who were full or partial owners of their practices and those who were nonowners (Boukus, Cassil and O'Malley, 2009; Leigh, Tancredi and Kravitz, 2009). Therefore, the association between practice ownership and pro-

Figure 8.2
Adjusted Associations Between Practice Organizational Model and Physician Professional Satisfaction

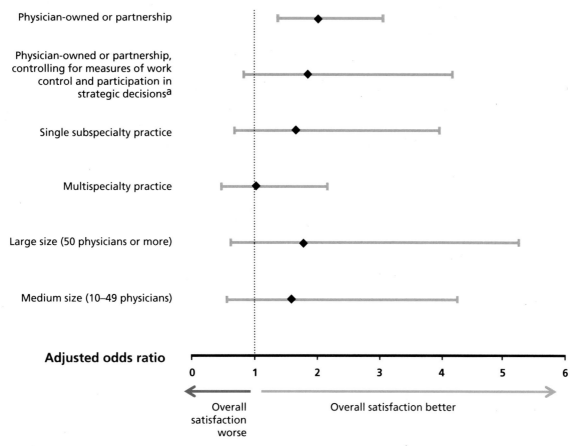

NOTES: Each estimate represents the effect of the corresponding practice model, relative to a comparison group. For practice ownership, the comparison group is "Hospital or corporate-owned"; for practice specialty, the comparison group is "Primary care"; and for size, the comparison group is "Small size (9 physicians or fewer)." Each odds ratio is adjusted for all other variables in the figure. 95-percent confidence intervals account for clustering of observations within practices. Statistically significant associations are highlighted by the use of colored confidence intervals: red for factors associated with worse satisfaction and green for factors associated with better satisfaction.
a Estimate additionally adjusted for opportunities to participate in strategic decisions and work control rating.
RAND *RR439-8.2*

fessional satisfaction (which was not a clear theme emerging from our qualitative analyses) requires confirmation in a nationally representative sample prior to serving as a guide for policy.

Figure 8.3
Adjusted Associations Between Aspects of Physicians' Autonomy, Work Control, and Difficulties Meeting Patient Needs—*Within Hospital- or Corporate-Owned Practices Only*

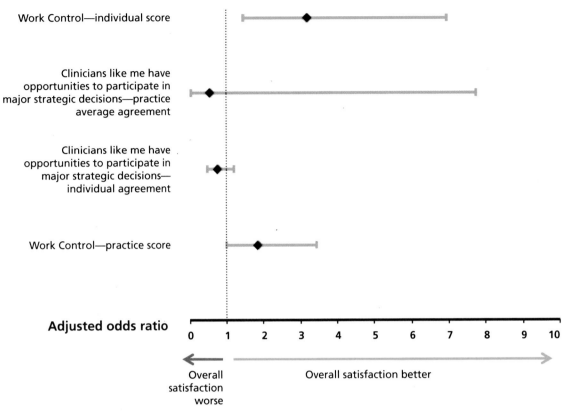

NOTES: Each estimate represents the effect of a one-point increase in the corresponding continuous score or agreeing or strongly agreeing with the corresponding statement among physicians who work in hospital- or corporate-owned practices. Effects are adjusted for practice size and specialty, as well as for individual response tendency. 95-percent confidence intervals account for clustering of observations within practices. Statistically significant associations are highlighted by the use of colored confidence intervals: red for factors associated with worse satisfaction and green for factors associated with better satisfaction.
RAND *RR439-8.3*

CHAPTER NINE

Practice Leadership

Overview of Findings

Among the practices we studied, practice leadership affected physician professional satisfaction in two main ways.

First, professional satisfaction was higher when physicians and their clinical colleagues reported that their values were well aligned with those of their leaders. Values alignment was especially important concerning approaches to clinical care. Some physicians reported that having leaders with clinical experience (either as physicians or other types of front-line clinical staff) enhanced the sense of values alignment between practice leaders and practicing physicians.

Second, physicians reported better professional satisfaction when practice leadership took a balanced approach to new practicewide initiatives, maintaining physician professional autonomy when possible.

Quantitative analyses of physician survey results also revealed alignment between leadership and physicians as a statistically significant predictor of better professional satisfaction. Similarly, scores on a "Facilitative leadership" scale (on which respondents rate their leaders' promotion of constructive change and an enjoyable workplace environment) and greater perceived respect from practice leaders were significantly associated with better professional satisfaction.

Qualitative Findings

Values Alignment with Practice Leadership

Physicians expressed satisfaction when they perceived that the organizational leadership shared the same values as they did, especially from a clinical standpoint. For example, the following physician explained how he valued having a practice leader who was a respected clinician and who listened carefully to the clinical rationale for an exception to guidelines:

> [Our practice leader] ... probably makes most of the decisions after evaluating costs and evidence-based medicine. ... So, for example, we have steroid injections and the lubricant injections and ... from a cost-effective standpoint ... maybe the steroid injection is the way to go. ... And so [our practice leader] actually asked me about that, ... and I told him, "Well, my patient population is a little different. I see teenagers, 30's, 40's, 50-year olds with degenerative knees, weekend warriors that may have a little bit of arthritis, and I've seen a therapeutic benefit when I [perform lubricant injections]. Yes, it's more expensive, but ... I

think doing a steroid injection in that age population may be detrimental to their cartilage and their meniscus." He thought about it and he said, "Okay, just make your decisions wisely." So he hasn't stopped me from using it. He could have easily have said, "Well, we're going to save the clinic $1,000, [so] no more [lubricant]." [But] he didn't do that. ... I think he's very, very reasonable.

—orthopedic surgeon

The advantage of having leaders with clinical experience was not limited to leaders who were physicians. As the following physician explained, practice leaders from other clinical fields, by "knowing what it's like" to be a front-line clinician, earned respect:

I think [satisfaction] does stem from the center manager, ... and most of our center managers have been with [the practice] for a long time. They may have started as medical records clerks, or front desk clerks, and just stayed and worked their way up. And so they know what it's like to be a medical records person, and now they're a center manager.

—obstetrician/gynecologist

Conversely, physicians in multiple practice models expressed dissatisfaction with practice leadership when there was a sense that leaders did not share their values concerning patient care. In some instances, this lack of values alignment was equated with having leaders who lacked, or had lost touch with, the direct patient care experience:

The dictatorship is coming from nonphysicians, and that's not good. ... I find that at the hospital, ... it's amazing how the administration determines how you'll deliver health care, and no matter how you try and influence that, as a medical staff, usually there's so much push from the top: "This is how we're going to do things." ... And we really struggle with things like that, where the administration, who don't do health care, are telling you how it's going to happen. They don't understand the intricacies of some of the things that we have to do as a physician.

—obstetrician/gynecologist

I'm a little worried that we're getting a dichotomy in medicine [with] people that are full-time administrators that really don't practice medicine anymore. ... Being in administration, I can tell you that my administrative jobs have always been less stressful than patient-care jobs. I can understand why people want a career in administrative medicine, but [in] 100-percent administrative medicine, you do lose touch, after a while, with what's going on the front lines with patients every day ... if you don't see people with medical problems and people that are very poor and can't afford health care and you have to try to figure out [how to help them].

—orthopedic surgeon

Balancing Leadership Initiatives with Physician Autonomy

Physicians described the variation in the way in which initiatives or mandates from practice leadership were implemented and how these approaches affected physician satisfaction.

Respondents valued flexibility when practice leaders implemented new initiatives while preserving physicians' freedom to make locally relevant decisions:

> Our medical director met with us very regularly. We had our consultants come in as we were looking at this new model that we were doing, and we met weekly for probably four months, it seemed. ... But it wasn't like a dictatorship that [said], "This is what you're going to do." [Instead, our practice leader said]: "Here's what we need to do. ... You craft it the way you want. I'm going to give you the tools to do it.".... He's been very, very highly involved, and I think that's good, but not as a micromanager, either.
>
> —manager of a multispecialty practice

Physicians reported appreciating clear explanations when new initiatives required new limits on their autonomy. As one leader of a large, multispecialty practice explained, preserving physician autonomy where it mattered most (e.g., picking compatible colleagues and staff) allowed practice leaders to focus their efforts to achieve a more uniform approach in areas where autonomy could detract from clinical care:

> I think that what [physicians are] least likely to give up control of is the particular staffing of their individual practices. You know, we involve physicians in ... recruiting additional providers, so that they feel that they're picking people that are compatible to work with them. ... What we have to move to more is standardizing our care protocols and plans, so that we're eliminating variation that's not beneficial, not adding value to what we do. And that can be a struggle because you know physicians, many have been trained with the art of medicine and, you know, individualizing care, and you have to have very deliberate conversations about, "Okay if this is best practice, and this is evidenced-based, why are you doing this differently, and how can you prove that you're adding value by doing that? And if you're not, then how do we get you to move away from that?" Very simple things like, you know, we're on an electronic medical record, and yet you have five physicians that are keeping separate paper files that then require additional staff in order to maintain those. And what value is being added to doing that? And so those are the tougher conversations, but they're conversations that you need to continue to have.
>
> —primary care physician, practice leader

Physicians also expressed dissatisfaction when practice leadership did not allow flexibility in implementing practice initiatives, especially when leadership was perceived as mandating broad solutions without fully understanding how problems varied from provider to provider:

> My concern with where we're going right now is that there's this tremendous pressure, economic pressure, to make people as productive as possible. ... There's this tendency ... when things aren't going well financially, to paint with this broad brush and sort of tell everybody, "You need to work harder." Well, you've got some people that are already working too hard. They ought to be being told to slow down a little bit because you can't do that and sustain it. But that's not what we do. We just say to everybody, "You need to see more patients." The terminology that's come up lately is "white space in your schedule." "Get rid of the white space." You know? So that's got to be a business thing of some kind. But so I think that can be very demoralizing to people, particularly people that are already pulling their share of the load or more than their share of the load, just to be told, "Well, you know,

you need to do more." Instead of ... finding the problems and dealing with the problems, [they are] ... sort of punishing everybody that's already ... trying to do the best they can.

—hematologist/oncologist

Quantitative Findings

Among physicians responding to our survey, 88 percent reported that their practice leaders respected them as professionals.

Congruent with qualitative findings, analyses of physician survey responses indicated that greater values alignment with practice leaders, high scores on the Facilitative Leadership scale, and greater perceived respect from practice leaders were associated with better overall professional satisfaction. These effects diminished in magnitude and lost statistical significance when ratings of leaders were aggregated to the practice level, possibly indicating that these constructs are not experienced equally among individuals within a given practice, that statistical power was limited at the practice level, or that residual response tendency bias may remain (despite our attempts to control for it). See Figure 9.1.

Comparison Between Current Findings and Previously Published Research

Our findings concerning the influence of practice leadership on professional satisfaction are similar to those from previous studies, conducted in a variety of specialties and settings, which have found better physician professional satisfaction when physicians share values with practice leaders and report that practice leaders recognize the value of their work (Linn, Yager, et al., 1985; Lewis et al., 1993a; Karsh, Beasley and Brown, 2010; Linzer et al., 2009).

**Figure 9.1
Adjusted Associations Between Physicians' Ratings of Practice Leaders and Overall Professional
Satisfaction**

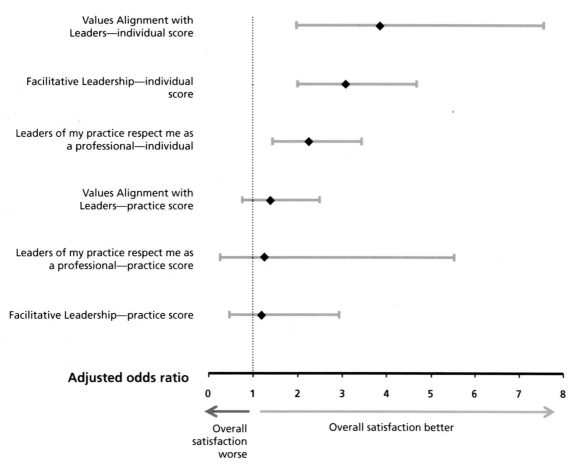

NOTES: Each estimate represents the effect of agreeing or strongly agreeing with the corresponding statement or a one-point increase in the corresponding continuous score. Effects are adjusted for practice size, specialty, and ownership; individual response tendency; and whether the respondent spends 10 percent or more of his or her working time doing management activities. 95-percent confidence intervals account for clustering of observations within practices. Statistically significant associations are highlighted by the use of colored confidence intervals: red for factors associated with worse satisfaction and green for factors associated with better satisfaction.
RAND RR439-9.1

CHAPTER TEN

Collegiality, Fairness, and Respect

Overview of Findings

Physicians' perceptions of collegiality, fairness, and respect were important determinants of professional satisfaction. In interviews, respondents reported four main areas in which these constructs operated: relationships with colleagues in the practice (including practice leadership), relationships with providers outside the practice, relationships with patients, and relationships with payers. Within the practice, frequent meetings with other physicians and allied health professionals (such as business meetings in physician partnerships) fostered greater collegiality. Some physicians who no longer co-owned their practices observed a decrease in interpersonal familiarity with their former partners when business meetings ceased, leading to lower overall morale.

Physicians reported limited but important specialty-specific frustrations with unfairness and disrespect when interacting with other providers. For surgeons, these concerns surfaced most prominently in arranging hospital call duties. For primary care physicians, interactions with other physicians were problematic when primary care physicians (and their staffs) were treated as subservient.

These findings generally were confirmed in quantitative analyses, and the influence of perceived respect from patients was an especially strong predictor of overall professional satisfaction.

Qualitative Findings

Below, we present the most commonly expressed themes describing the effects of collegiality, fairness, and respect on professional satisfaction. We start with relationships between colleagues within the practice and then proceed to relationships with providers outside the practice, with patients, and with payers.

Collegiality, Teamwork, and Respect Among Physicians and Staff Within Practices

Physicians in a variety of practice arrangement described the importance of being able to trust their colleagues with their patients. As one physician described, knowing that one's colleagues have a common practice style was a source of satisfaction:

> Number one, I think [it's important to be] giving your service to somebody else you know. You've been taking care of these patients for a week. Now, you're about to pass those patients off. I think, especially in really sick patients, when you've had end-of-life conversations and

have really developed relationships with families, you really like to think that you're going to be giving those patients to somebody who's very similar to you in the way that you practice, in the way that you talk to patients and families.

—hospitalist

Collaborative teamwork involving physicians and other practice staff was also reported as a source of professional satisfaction and a key contributor to the efficient allocation of work tasks. As one medical assistant described:

I've never been afraid to actually go up to any doctor and say, "I have this question about this patient." Or, "I have this concern about what's going on." ... We say, "We have this patient walking in. What do we do? This is the scenario." I've never had [a physician in this practice say], "No, I don't want to talk to you right now," or, "No, I can't take care of that." It's always, "What do you need?" I like that.

—medical assistant in a primary care practice

In [pediatrics], we really have started to leverage our [registered nurses] a lot, and it's been wonderful. The families have loved it. They get this consistent product. ... [The nurses] make sure that they get all these education pieces done and then let [the physicians] do the work that [they] do, so it's actually been really positive.

—practice administrator

In multispecialty practices, ease of collaboration between physicians in different specialties was a reported source of support:

Well that's one of the big advantages of a multispecialty group, ... that you have that immediate access. So, I get a lot of phone calls during the day from doctors. ... I think that we're able to serve as a resource for those people. But I'm also able to call people myself, and I do that.

—medical subspecialist

However, some physicians reported difficulty transitioning to forms of teamwork that did not have clear physician leadership. One physician described losing a sense of respect in a team that featured equal status among physicians and other staff members, even when physicians bore more personal risk:

I'm a little baffled by ... this whole egalitarian thing going on, where everyone is kind of at the same level, from front desk, to medical assistants, to nurses, to nurse practitioners, to docs. All the docs and nurse practitioners are called "providers" because it's the common denominator. ... I don't feel like it's really that respectful a place for a physician to work, because the physician, in my mind, is taking on tremendous risk. ... [It's] the same risk that any primary care doctor takes on. Risk of failure to diagnose. Risk of failure to timely diagnose. Risk of prescribing a medication with an adverse effect. ... There is this lack of the basic respect that ... it's the physician's license, and the physician's reputation, and the physician's risk.

—primary care physician

Respect from Practice Leaders

Satisfying collaboration among colleagues required support and communication from practice leaders, and physicians reported decreased satisfaction when these ingredients were lacking. In particular, they expressed a desire to have clear, straightforward explanations for why leaders reached their decisions, especially when they perceived these decisions as preventing successful teams from forming:

> I feel that something that gets lost ... [is] feeling appreciated by your organization. ... If we felt that [practice leaders] were more concerned about [the problems we see] and trying to fix them, we would feel more satisfied. ... If these issues with triage and stuff that could really be changed, ... we would feel more appreciated. So, we're not feeling very appreciated is what I'm saying, because things that we keep complaining about just aren't being fixed. ... We'll probably be happier if you just told us that the reason why we can't have a nurse is because we don't have enough money to hire a nurse. We would understand that, but we don't get [an explanation]. So we're sitting there like nobody cares about us not having a nurse.
>
> —primary care physician

The relationship between disrespect from practice leadership and professional dissatisfaction was not limited to large practices. As one physician described, these concerns were important among small, physician-led practices as well:

> There was a husband and wife and another doctor who were working together at another clinic in [name of city]. And they, to put it bluntly, sort of felt like they were getting shafted. They weren't really equal partners in the group, and they didn't have much control. And they thought, "This isn't how we want to practice. We don't like this environment." And so they started [name of clinic]. And their goal from very early on was to create a, sort of an egalitarian work environment, ... and that spirit really remains. ... [I started as] an employed physician, but I was invited to all the meetings. I was welcome and invited to speak up about stuff and really felt right from the get-go, like one of the gang. So that was a good feeling.
>
> —primary care physician

Regular Interpersonal Contact Can Foster Collegiality

Physicians, especially those in partnerships, described how their practice management meetings fostered collegiality with their physician colleagues. These meetings gave physicians a chance to get to know each other better, as a beneficial side effect of running a business:

> The physicians are very happy here. I mean, it seems like things work well. To get [approximately 40 physicians] to sit down and agree on anything, I don't know [how] they can do that, but they do, so that's pretty impressive there. And I think they're pretty careful about who they invite into a partnership here. They want to make sure they're of the same mindset of, "Hey, I want to be here a long time, I want to play well with others, I want to work in a productive nature, I want to make this the good life."
>
> —physician assistant

We had a clinic meeting over at the house the other day, and … my wife was listening upstairs, and afterwards she said, "It sounded like you were having so much fun, everybody laughing. What was going on down there?" … I hadn't thought of it until later, but, you know, she was thinking it sounded like it was a fun party.

—primary care physician

When partnerships were acquired by larger organizations, regular business meetings were no longer necessary. With the end of these meetings, some physicians expressed a desire to find a new reason to meet, to recover the collegiality they now missed. As one physician, whose partnership practice recently had been acquired by a hospital, explained:

We've got to find some way to get the physicians across the practice lines here within [the practice] meeting and interacting on a more regular basis. As a private group, we met once a month, and that was dinner, … and you talk, and there's a lot more to a meeting than just talking about business. … It's team building, and that's what I see is missing right now. I would like to see us … get back to some type of a monthly meeting.

—primary care physician

Relationships with Providers and Delivery Systems Outside the Practice
Physicians reported valuing collegial relationships with providers in other institutions, even when their institutions were competitors. As one physician described, maintaining such relationships was particularly important when competing practices shared a single hospital:

We had the [other institution] and [our practice], and I always felt really good that, from a political standpoint our administrations may have not gotten along, but clinically I felt like we were a cohesive department. We were supportive of each other, and it was nice because there was always somebody on call from our group and somebody on call from their group, and if you had a really hard case or you just needed some help, you knew there was somebody else that was available. … From a physician standpoint, I think that we all get along just fine, … [even though] there are some political undertones [between our institutions] that are not as positive.

—pediatrician

Conversely, physicians described how perceiving disrespectful behavior by physicians in other practices and other specialties could be a source of frustration. In some cases, payer rules contributed to these unwelcome behaviors:

One of the things about being an internist that really grates on my nerves is that everything rolls down to the internist. So, just to give you an example, I had a patient two days ago. It's 4:00 in the afternoon. I have a patient who is seeing an ophthalmologist who has papilledema, and the ophthalmologist wasn't internal [to our practice], was an outsider, called me and says, "I think the patient has pseudotumor cerebri. Needs to see a neuro-ophthalmologist, but they won't see the patient unless they have an MRI of their brain, their orbits, and a lumbar puncture, and can you please arrange that?" I'm not a secretary, but I ended up having to, you know, corral my staff to do it, and it was very disruptive because it had to be done, you know, ASAP. … I don't see why an ophthalmologist can't have their staff do that. ... Some of that is driven by the health insurances. ... [For] the MRI, the approval had to come from the primary [care physician], so ... we get stuck doing things that are not necessarily things that we order.

—primary care physician

For surgeons in particular, fairness and respect concerning hospitals' expectations of call coverage were reported as having important effects on professional satisfaction. As the manager of a surgical practice explained:

I sense a great deal of frustration with the call issues. What's happened in this area is the hospital is a regional referral center, and so a lot of the outside hospitals just send patients here. ... Some of those urologists [from the outside hospital] actually live up here. So, our doctors are driving by their friend's house on the way to take care of their [friend's] patients, you know. So, that's the type of frustration they have. That's something we really need to address. So far, the hospital has been very resistant to any sort of pay-for-call discussions, but somehow we need to deal with that. As reimbursements drop for physicians, their ability to sustain a call schedule while taking care of their own patients the day after [a call has become] much more difficult. They don't have the luxury to say, "Well, tomorrow I'll take the day off because I was up all night."

—practice manager

As a surgeon in another practice described, resigning from a hospital call system perceived as unfair improved professional satisfaction:

The [call structure] has changed recently, which has been wonderful. So my partner and I, since we do primarily [specialty surgery], we basically did not feel like we were gaining much from being on call here at the hospital for the ER, and so we pulled out of the ER call schedule about a year and a half ago, which was a huge satisfier in my life. They restructured the call program over at the hospital, [and] they're having the trauma surgeons now cover the ER call, which made the trauma surgeons happy because they were finally getting some cases, which they needed, and we aren't covering the ER all weekend and seeing a bunch of patients who don't pay anything, which is what we were doing.

—general surgeon

Respect from Patients

Few physicians in our sample reported feeling disrespected by their patients. However, some interviewees reported interactions with patients that implied disrespect for their training and credentials, and these interactions were sources of professional dissatisfaction. In general, physicians tended to attribute such disrespect to the influence of third parties, like the popular media. For example, the following physician reported being taken aback by patients' requests to interview him before deciding whether to choose him as their doctor:

The news is [telling patients] to demand more and more. For one thing, I've had some patients come in and say they want to interview me before [having their first appointment]. ... I just haven't been able to handle that. I just say, "If that's the way you feel, you need to go talk to another doctor." ... But that's what they tell them on Good Morning America, so I'm sure that's going to be a big thing in the future. People are going to interview you to see if [they] want you for [their] doctor.

—primary care physician

Respect from Payers

Physicians spanning the specialties and practice models in our study described a sense that certain tools payers use (e.g., prior authorizations) were disrespectful to them, especially when they interfered with good patient care. As a result of these tools, relationships with patients were also stressed in some instances:

> I think there is a lot more interference, not so much from the government, [but] from insurance companies, trying to cut corners. I will see a patient for diabetes and come out here and write a prescription, and they'll say the insurance company won't cover this. Call this number and spend 20 minutes waiting. … You get one number, you wait and wait and wait and wait, and it's increasing encroachment on the patient-physician relationship, second guessing the things that we order. I think that probably underlined the thing I find most objectionable … a seeming lack of respect for doctors that seemed to be there before and now just it seems to be eroding in the present system.

—primary care physician

Quantitative Findings

Among physicians responding to our survey, nearly all reported feeling respected by their patients and colleagues. The majority also reported that outside reviewers rarely questioned their professional judgments. Approximately two in five primary care physicians reported easy access to "curbside" consults. See Table 10.1.

Consistent with qualitative findings, higher scores on measures of practice team functioning ("relationship infrastructure" and "sensemaking") were associated with better professional satisfaction. These relationships were stronger at the individual level than at the practice level, possibly indicating that individuals within a given practice did not experience these constructs equally (or that residual response tendency bias may remain, despite our attempts to control for it). Also consistent with qualitative findings, fairness of compensation was a statistically significant predictor of greater overall satisfaction.

Despite the low number of physicians reporting that their patients did not respect them, respect from patients was a significant predictor of professional satisfaction—more so than indicators of respect from payers and colleagues. See Figure 10.1.

Comparison Between Current Findings and Previously Published Research

Similar to the current study, previous research, conducted among physicians in a variety of practice settings, has found that physicians who perceived good working relationships with other physicians (including perceptions of teamwork) and with staff in their practice were also

Table 10.1
Responses to Survey Questions About Respect from Patients and Colleagues

Item	Percentage
Responding "Agree" or "Strongly agree" to the following:	
My patients respect me as a professional	96
Co-workers in my practice respect me as a professional	94
Outside reviewers rarely question my professional judgments	63
Responding "Always/most of the time" to the following:	
When clinically appropriate, how often is it easy to obtain a doctor-to-doctor ("curbside") consult from a specialist in lieu of referring the patient?	42

more likely to report being satisfied with their jobs and their overall careers than were those who did not report good working relationships with other physicians (Williams et al., 1999; Linzer et al., 2000; Stoddard et al., 2001; Linn et al., 1986; Karsh, Beasley and Brown, 2010; Linzer et al., 2009; Cydulka and Korte, 2008; Lewis et al., 1993b).

In the current study, perceived respect from patients was associated with professional satisfaction. To our knowledge, no previously published study has specifically examined the relationship between perceived respect from patients (which was an original survey item) and professional satisfaction.

Figure 10.1
Adjusted Associations Between Measures of Practice Collegiality, Respect, and Overall Professional Satisfaction

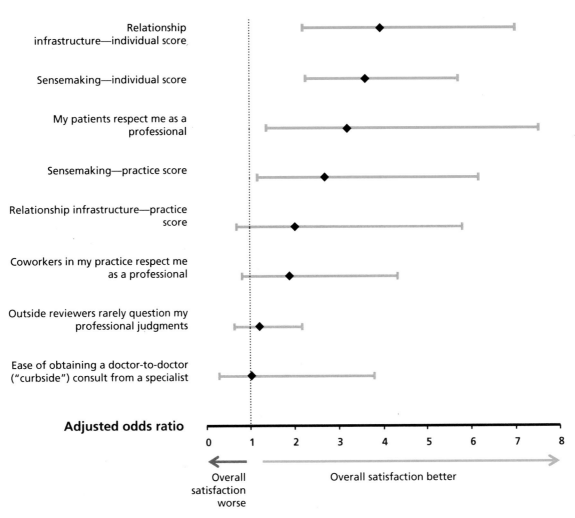

NOTES: Each estimate represents the effect of agreeing or strongly agreeing with the corresponding statement or a one-point increase in the corresponding continuous score. Odds ratios are adjusted for practice size, specialty, and ownership, as well as for individual response tendency. 95-percent confidence intervals account for clustering of observations within practices. Statistically significant associations are highlighted by the use of colored confidence intervals: red for factors associated with worse satisfaction and green for factors associated with better satisfaction.

RAND RR439-10.1

CHAPTER ELEVEN

Work Quantity and Pace

Overview of Findings

Physicians, clinical staff, and practice leaders commonly reported challenges stemming from the quantity and pace of physician work. Especially in primary care specialties, physicians described how pressure to provide greater quantities of services effectively limited the time and attention they could spend with each individual patient, detracting from the quality of care in some cases.

Some of the physicians we interviewed had joined practices in which payment did not rely on the number of patients seen, but in doing so, they reported accepting lower incomes. Others reported that improvement strategies adapted from other industries (e.g., lean improvement techniques) had improved patient flow, yielding a more reasonable work pace and less time pressure.

Importantly, a smaller number of physicians and practices reported that dissatisfaction (and worries about practice sustainability) could also stem from insufficient work quantity. These concerns were most commonly articulated by the surgeons in our study.

Quantitative analyses of survey responses generally corroborated these findings, with time pressure being a strong predictor of overall professional dissatisfaction.

Qualitative Findings

Excessive Time Pressure Worsens Physician Professional Satisfaction

Managers of primary care practices commonly described excessive work volume, coupled with insufficient time, as a source of physician frustration:

> [One problem is] being overpaneled, maybe. Not being able to meet the demand of what the patients' needs are. I know that [physicians] feel as though they want to do a little bit more face-to-face time or be able to call a patient, rather than have a nurse do it. They want to have that empathy or that caring part. Sometimes I feel they get frustrated that they aren't able to have enough time to be able to do that. I know they get frustrated when it comes to that.
>
> —manager of a primary care practice

Another practice manager described visit lengths approaching seven minutes, as local primary care practices attempted to respond to a perceived shortage of primary care providers:

I think, in primary care, we're looking at a shortage. ... We're proud of the fact that we separate ourselves from, literally, the seven-minute visits. In town, that's kind of the issue … primary care physicians feel squeezed in other organizations. They feel like they don't have enough time with the patients. Their panels are too large. They're working too much, and I think that's pretty standard for any primary care population.

—practice manager, primary care

Even outside office visits, the work required to maintain large patient panels in primary care generated stress:

[My panel size is] about 3,200 and I'm actively trying to decrease it. ... It's hard because, you know, all those people are calling. They may not be seeing you, but they're still calling for refills. They're still calling [with] questions, and you still have to follow up on their labs that may be coming in and make [medication] adjustments and things like that. So, it's a lot more paperwork or [EHR] work.

—primary care physician

When a practice's main source of revenue was physician fee-for-service billings, some observed that financial dependence on physician work volume worsened time pressure for physicians, relative to clinical staff, whose work was less important to practice finances. Although not limited to primary care, this finding was particularly prominent among the primary care practices in our sample:

Whenever there seems to be economic stress, it seems like we're sort of the money makers for this place. I think we generate a lot of income. And so … your nutritionists, I don't know how they're reimbursed, not very well, can spend an hour with a patient. We get 20 minutes, come hell or high water, no matter what it is. And that's true across the board. Everybody gets more time than [physicians] do, partly because our time is more valuable.

—primary care physician

Especially in primary care, some physicians described an expanding volume of work per visit, further exacerbating the perception of time pressure. For example, one physician described how additional services, such as medication reconciliation, although beneficial, led to even more work per visit:

I guess it's the wave of the future is to be able to see more patients in a shorter amount of time. ... I just don't think a 15-minute visit is remotely feasible. I think it's ridiculous that they expect … me to update their health maintenance, reconcile their medications, and see them for their problem. ... And then, usually, when you update something, it suddenly gets them to talk about that other thing. They're like, "Oh, you're really in for a sinus infection. We just updated your [medications], and you told me you're not taking your antidepressants." Now, we're talking about depression.

—primary care physician

When time pressure led to sufficient discomfort, some physicians left their practices, especially when they perceived the time pressure was a threat to the quality of care. As one physician explained, time pressure was especially acute when patients had greater language needs and higher acuity, leading her to leave a previous practice:

> The unrelenting pace of patient care, especially in the setting that I was in, where 70 percent of our clinic visits were [language] interpreted, ... with 15- and 20-minute visits for people who avoid seeking health care until they have serious problems, not only led to innumerable long hours, but also was an error waiting to happen. You know, there isn't time to ask all the questions that need to be asked, to do all the informed consent that needs to be done. There just isn't the time. And you do your best every single day, but you see things, you see near misses that you can do nothing about, because the system has no more capacity to reach further, and the system has no more time to help those people. So [I left the practice], after years and years of that frustration and the risk, knowing that your license could be in jeopardy at any point, even though you're trying 120 percent to do the best by everybody, because you can't catch everything at that pace.
>
> —primary care physician

Providers who switched practice models to reduce time pressure reported better satisfaction and better perceived ability to provide high-quality care, even if their salaries were lower as a result:

> [At another local primary care practice,] I think their salaries are probably a little higher, but the bean counters tell them how many people they've got to see. I know in one group, if you don't make your quota every day, they dock your pay. So, if you're really caught where you got a tough patient who has an issue you can't quite decide, or needs counseling and is crying and their child is five, whatever, you know, if they know they're going to dock your pay if you spend a little more time being humanly kind, that's different than, "If I don't see another patient, maybe some patient will have to wait." [Here,] we're under ... our own control. We decide what we want to do. I think that appeals a lot to me and other people.
>
> —primary care physician

> The biggest difference [between my current practice and my old practice] is that I have time to talk to people. I have time to get a real history. I have time to do a physical exam. ... I find out about a patient's context and what may be a barrier to them getting that medicine, whether that's an unsupportive partner or that maybe their own job is as hectic as my last job was, and so they just don't have the time to find a pharmacy that's going to be convenient for them to get to, or to go for a mammogram or to get an ultrasound. Some barrier is there, and I just didn't have the time before to assess that, and now I do. I have time to listen and explain.
>
> —primary care physician

Work-Life Balance

Separate from time pressure, physicians in a variety of specialties and practice models described a tension between fulfilling their patient care duties, keeping their length of working day manageable, and achieving acceptable work-life balance:

There's a number of things I'd like, but one of them goes back to the quality of life. I think our last patient's at 5:20. No one here leaves before 6:30, and no one's work is done before 6:30. I think that [it would be good] to somehow shave the number of patients that we're required to see a day so that it's more of a 9:00 to 5:00 in the office job. Now, not one of us went into medicine expecting 9:00 to 5:00, yet as we've grown, lots of us have young families. You want more time with that. I'd like to be able to see less patients to provide more comprehensive care, because I do feel rushed. I do feel like, trying to make ends meet, trying to take care of my panel, I do shortchange people on time, and I'd like to not have to do that.

—primary care physician

However, primary care physicians in several practices noted that the advent of hospitalists had improved their work-life balance substantially:

Call's gone through quantum shift for me. Call used to be the worst part of my life. It was awful. It was just miserable because I've still got horrors of [my colleague] in the emergency room calling me at 2:00 in the morning. ... So I go at 3:00, be back at 5:00 having worked up a chest pain with a heart attack or maybe a diverticulitis or something like that. I'm not complaining, I'm just telling you what it was. ... Crawled back in bed maybe at 5:00, woke up at 6:00 and went in and did a full day in the office. Total misery. I didn't realize it, because I was 40, and I could do it. Now, fast forward 20 years, I never get a phone call, I do not have to go to the emergency room, I don't have to make rounds in the hospital. ... I think it changed when the hospitalists came along.

—primary care physician

In other practices, shared priorities among physician colleagues enabled work-life balance to be prioritized over additional income:

Well, I think from a physician point of view, one of the things about our practice is [that] we try and have a good balance of quality of life, lifestyle, and compensation. [If] you don't work, you don't get paid, so the more time you take off, the lower your income is going to be. And so ... if someone comes in and they're wanting to make an absolute fortune in a short period of time, then this is probably not the place for them to be. But if they want to have a reasonable quality of life, family time, time to enjoy the occasional sunny day we have here ... , they're much more likely to be happy with this kind of group.

—primary care physician

Practice Improvement Strategies to Manage Workload

A small number of primary care physicians within our study, both in small and large practices, reported having engaged in practice improvement strategies to better manage patient flow and reduce time pressure. These physicians described lean improvement strategies, adapted from other industries, as being helpful.[1] The following physician describes how, despite initial skepti-

---

[1]   "Lean" strategies seek to redesign processes for greater efficiency by standardizing work (as appropriate), eliminating inefficiencies, and tracking progress toward goals. A recent study found that lean methods in cardiac units were associated with lower mortality rates from acute myocardial infarction (McConnell et al., 2013).

cism about "lean" practices, such as labeling office supplies in a uniform manner, this redesign strategy ultimately improved his satisfaction with practice:

> So, the whole … thing is built on the Toyota model, you know, the lean collaborative. You've heard about these things, and it makes sense, but you never [quite believe it]—I mean it is very tedious to label everything. … [But after] you put the whole thing together, it's very difficult [not] to think, "Well, why didn't I do it before?" … I'm feeling a lot better. You know, I'm taking more care of my health now. … [Before lean], when you're in this black hole, you feel like you're sucked in. You feel like you're trapped. You feel like there's nowhere to go. … It's like you're on a treadmill, and if you stop, you fall. Now [after lean redesign], you have room to wiggle a little bit.
>
> —primary care physician

Too Few Patients or Concern About Practice Sustainability

Although fewer physicians reported having too few patients, insufficient work quantity was another potential source of dissatisfaction. While this was not a universal viewpoint, multiple surgeons in our study described greater case volume as a driver of better satisfaction. As one surgeon reported, a perceived scarcity of cases among local surgeons could be a source of anxiety:

> I think a lot of [satisfaction] has to do with how busy they are. Referral sources, the types of cases they're doing. There's only a certain number of cases. We can't make more cases, and with [a given] number of surgeons, if someone gets more cases, that means someone's going to get less. There's no [new cases] to fill in someone who's losing cases, so I think the busier you are, and generating a good income stream, then you tend to be happier. If you're not as busy, then you're not as happy in general.
>
> —general surgeon

Uneven demand also raised concern about practice sustainability. These concerns were expressed most often by physicians who were owners or partners in their practices:

> We definitely need to be busier. Every year we go through this. It's really busy in the winter—as a pediatrician, you know—and then it slows down in the summer. We still have to pay the mortgage every month, and we have electricity every month, and it's hard to balance that with [high demand] in the winter [but] nothing in the summer. So it would be nice to be productive year round and have like a steady stream of patients instead of this ebb and flow.
>
> —pediatrician

Quantitative Findings

Among physicians responding to our survey, three in five reported having adequate time with their patients. Only one in five reported that work rarely encroached on their personal lives, but three in four were satisfied with their vacation and call. Nearly all were "full time" workers (>30 work-hours/week), with a median of 2,300 work hours per year (with an interquartile range of 1,840 to 2,800). About one-half reported feeling pressure to attract and retain patients, and one in four reported a chaotic practice atmosphere. Depending on the type of patient visit, between 30 and 40 percent of physicians reported having insufficient time to provide the services patients needed. See Table 11.1.

Congruent with our qualitative findings, analyses of survey data revealed that having sufficient time with patients was a statistically significant determinant of professional satisfaction. A generally chaotic practice atmosphere was also a significant predictor of dissatisfaction, and there were trends toward greater overall satisfaction when the work-life balance was better (e.g., less work encroachment on personal life). Full-time (defined as 30 hours or more per week) versus part-time work was not significantly associated with overall satisfaction. This result may reflect physicians having already made choices to pursue their preferred work-life balance, with few physicians feeling "trapped" in full-time positions or vice versa. See Figure 11.1.

Table 11.1
Responses to Survey Questions About Work Quantity and Pace

Item	Percentage
Responding "Agree" or "Strongly agree" to the following:	
"I have adequate time to spend with my patients during their office visits"	60
"Work rarely encroaches on my personal life"	20
"I am satisfied with the amount of vacation time I have in my current job"	74
"The amount of call I am required to take is not excessive"	73
"Time pressures keep me from developing good patient relationships"	19
Reporting the following:	
Full-time worker (30 hours or more per week)	95
A lot or a moderate amount of pressure to attract and retain patients	47
Chaotic practice atmosphere	25
Average time allocated to complete physical/consultation for a new patient	
50% to 100% of time needed	33
<50% of time needed	9
Average time allocated for a routine follow-up visit with an established patient	
50% to 100% of time needed	24
<50% of time needed	5
Average time allocated for an urgent care or acute visit	
50% to 100% of time needed	23
<50% of time needed	10

Comparison Between Current Findings and Previously Published Research

Similar to our study, findings from a study of family practitioners and internists in New York and the Upper Midwest (An et al., 2009; Linzer et al., 2009), as well as from a study of academic and clinical faculty at one academic medical center (Linn, Yager, et al., 1985), indicated that greater time pressure to perform clinical duties was associated with lower physician satisfaction.

Figure 11.1
Adjusted Associations Between Measures of Work Quantity, Work Pace, and Overall Professional Satisfaction

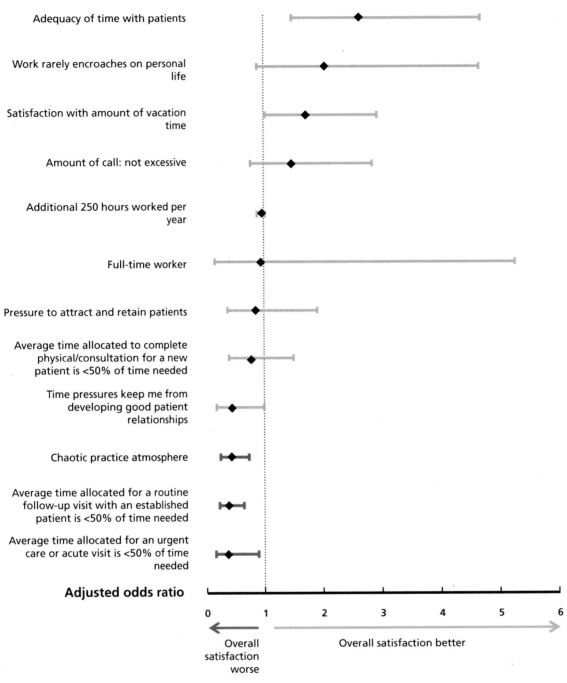

NOTES: Each estimate represents the effect of agreeing or strongly agreeing with the corresponding statement, reporting the corresponding category of time pressure or chaos, being a full-time worker (30 hours or more per week), or reporting a chaotic practice atmosphere. Odds ratios are adjusted for practice size, specialty, and ownership, as well as for individual response tendency. 95-percent confidence intervals account for clustering of observations within practices. Statistically significant associations are highlighted by the use of colored confidence intervals: red for factors associated with worse satisfaction and green for factors associated with better satisfaction.
RAND *RR439-11.1*

CHAPTER TWELVE

Work Content, Allied Health Professionals, and Support Staff

Overview of Findings

In general, physicians described better satisfaction when their work content matched their training and dissatisfaction when they were required to perform work that other staff could perform—especially when they sensed that the content of their work was being dictated to them. Specific types of satisfying work varied by specialty and by individual, but some patterns emerged. For example, many primary care physicians appreciated providing care that was continuous, including inpatient care. Some of these physicians missed caring for hospitalized patients, expressing concern about losing their skills in inpatient medicine when hospitalists cared for their inpatients. Among surgeons, some expressed a desire to develop expertise in a specific niche within their field.

Working with adequate numbers of well-trained, trusted, and capable allied health professionals and support staff was a key contributor to greater physician professional satisfaction. Support from such staff enabled physicians to achieve a more desirable mix of work content. Several study participants appreciated having long-term working relationships with allied health professionals and support staff, with some such relationships spanning decades. This theme was corroborated in quantitative analyses of physician survey responses, which revealed that greater staff stability (i.e., lower turnover) was a significant predictor of better overall professional satisfaction.

Qualitative Findings

Work Content

Physicians in a wide range of specialties and all practice models included in this study described deriving satisfaction from delivering patient care that matched their level of training. The following orthopedic surgeon contrasted his current experiences, in which he delegated work that did not require his specific training to his staff, with his experiences in a prior practice, where less delegation was possible:

> I have a scheduling [assistant]. I have a [physician assistant], and she has a nurse. So, a lot of that stuff that a lot of doctors do is fairly heavily delegated from me. … For a doctor to be productive in the current environment, he or she needs to practice at the top of their license. For me, that's deciding who needs surgery and [operating] in the operating room, and seeing you in the hospital, making decisions, making rounds, and all that. Other than that, [the remaining work is] not the top of my license. Changing dressings, taking out staples,

writing discharge orders, ... I don't do that anymore. ... It goes back to why I left the first group, ... they get mired in this paperwork, ... which, for me, was very dissatisfying, so I hired people to do it. ... I think if most people would do that, they would be happier and more financially satisfied.

—orthopedic surgeon

Similarly, the following physician felt that much of her work was actually secretarial, but she did not see a clear way to delegate this work to others within her practice. These factors contributed to significant dissatisfaction, particularly since they interfered with her ability to provide direct patient care:

[Physicians] get 20 minutes [per visit], come hell or high water, no matter what it is. And that's true across the board. Everybody [else] gets more time than we do, partly because our time is more valuable. ... And yet, interestingly enough, I think we do a lot of crap. We're paid to do ... a lot of secretarial work that seems to me other people could be doing. ... If I just had to see my patients [without having to do this secretarial work], I'm going to take care of them in a way I think is good. The job would be almost delightful.

—primary care physician

Specific Components of Work Content

In addition to broadly describing how being able to specify the content of their work was an important component of physician satisfaction, physicians and providers in this survey cited a number of more-specific components of their work, which were important. Some components were noted by physicians of all specialties, while other components were more specific to the physicians' specialties.

Continuity of Care

Physicians and providers saw value in continuity of care, both for the purposes of medical management and because they derived enjoyment from being able to know their patients and developing relationships with them over time. In light of increasing use of hospitalists, from an intellectual standpoint, physicians missed the ability to make management decisions in a variety of settings (e.g., inpatient and outpatient):

Personally, the breadth of primary care internal medicine was [appealing] when I went into it as a resident. And so, seeing some of the opportunities that were inherent in providing longitudinal primary care, it's been difficult to see those taken away [by hospitalists], primarily, it seems, because of economic reasons. ... I still hear patients saying how much they miss having one person providing continuity of care. While I could go and visit them if I had time in the hospital, I don't have the opportunity ... to actually see them and be a part of the management in the hospital.

—primary care physician

There was concern, particularly among physicians, that newer models of care might preclude their ability to personally provide continuous patient care:

[I worry that] implementing the team-based approach means I'm going see the patients less. ... It's going to be more, you know, didactic and "check the box" and get the patient out and figure out a plan for the team to take care of them and then step back and let the team take care of them. ... Somehow, nobody is really looking at that other physician satisfaction piece that says, "We enjoy the relationships we have with our patients and [helping with] the ups and downs of their lives." And we're going to have to figure out a way to replace some of that when we step back and let others kind of take care of our patients.

—primary care physician

Hospital Care for Primary Care Physicians

One important factor in the content of physicians' work, particularly for primary care physicians, was whether they saw patients in the hospital. This became particularly relevant following the increased use of hospitalists for inpatient care. While many practices reported that it did not make financial sense to continue seeing their hospitalized patients, given their small numbers and the amount of time it required, many physicians also described enjoying that aspect of patient care. Practices had found various solutions to this issue, with some giving up hospital care altogether. For the following physician, having hospitalists and not having to go to the hospital was positive overall, but the cost was missing important aspects of her patients' care:

I do miss ... the intensity of taking care of [hospitalized] patients. It's like the full picture, and you're missing part of the picture [by not caring for patients in the hospital]. But, as far as satisfaction, it was very inefficient. ... I would go to my first job, be in the hospital in the morning. Then my second job would be here. Then sometimes you have to go back to your first job again. Then you'd be on call and working the first job. So, from a satisfaction standpoint, ... it's much better not to have to do that. But, part of me misses [the hospital].

—primary care physician

Other practices devised hybrid solutions:

There's been talk back and forth over the years about [whether a] hospitalist system [could] absorb our inpatient needs. Although, there's this ongoing tension in the group ... [because] we like taking care of our own patients. We like practicing inpatient medicine. And at the same time, ... if we didn't have to do it, maybe we'd be able to generate more outpatient clinical income and be yet happier again. But the current inpatient strategy is that ... we admit our own patients, and then the doctor who is on for the week as the practice hospitalist from our group takes over that patient care. ... So, we essentially provide our own internal hospitalist coverage. ... For those of us who don't have a lot of patients who are sick and hospitalized, it gives us good hospital experience on an ongoing basis. So we get to continue to keep our foot sort of in the door and keep our hospital skills up.

—primary care physician

Even in practices where primary care physicians continued to practice inpatient medicine, interviewees described a sense that phasing out this practice was inevitable:

When that whole hospitalist movement came in, ... we really were ingrained in the hospital in inpatient care and call, and we really liked that part of our practice. So we kind of fought [our practice headquarters] when they wanted to put in the hospitalists and take us out of the hospital. We bargained for a hybrid model where we have hospitalists, but they don't cover our patients all the time. ... As time has gone on, and we've gotten older, it's [become] harder to take those weekend night calls and come back and work on Monday and all that. So we're actually kind of moving more toward hiring more hospitalists and letting some of the internists out of the hospital work.

—primary care physician

Subspecialty Niches for Surgeons

Multiple surgeons reported that it was important for them to develop deep expertise within a niche. For example, the following orthopedic surgeon described choosing his current practice because, in part, he was able to achieve a focused case mix, accumulating greater case volume and technical expertise:

I think one of the big factors [in choosing this practice] was that I would be able to practice 80 to 90 percent [of the time] in what I was trained to do, whereas [in my earlier practice, I was] kind of just doing everything. ... Here, really, my niche has been sports medicine and shoulder reconstruction. So, ... I haven't had to do a carpal tunnel, and I haven't had to do some elective foot procedure or anything like that, because I have ... foot, ankle, and hand guys ... here. So I am able to practice really what I want to do. I think that's really important simply because there are some folks that are just naturally talented and really, really gifted, but surgeons are technicians and you get better with experience.

—orthopedic surgeon

Allied Health Professionals and Support Staff

In general, physicians reported that working with allied health professionals and support staff who performed key tasks—such as handling incoming messages and fulfilling patient requests that did not require a physician's attention—could make important contributions to better professional satisfaction:

I think that we would benefit from having more clinical staff between the doctors and the medical assistants. ... Having other clinical staff to make decisions, like all these phone calls that come in: "Can this person refill their nasal spray?" We have yet to find a way to really take physicians out of that equation. I think that would free up a lot of time. ... A lot of us feel sort of awash in information, ... and just having some help managing that flow of information [would be helpful].

—primary care physician

Some physicians noted the importance of being able to know and trust the allied health professionals and support staff with whom they worked (as with knowing and trusting the other physicians with whom they shared patients). When there was less trust, physicians were also less comfortable with delegating tasks:

I think it's always harder when you're talking to [an allied health professional] you don't know. ... It's hard for you to know how much you can trust their judgment. ... Whereas [with] nurses that I know well enough that if they say, "Hey, this is what's going on, but I have a good handle on it. You don't need to come see them." I'm totally comfortable with that. [But] sometimes it might be something as minor as getting a phone call about a blood pressure and you're kind of like, "Eh, I'm going to go up and see that patient because I don't know you, and I don't know if you're assessing the patient the way I would."

—hospitalist

Long-standing relationships between physicians, allied health professionals, and support staff were described as important to developing trust and good communication. When new staffing models disrupted these relationships, some physicians expressed significant anxiety. For example, one physician who had worked with a particular medical assistant (MA) exclusively for other a decade and who was now transitioning to a shared-MA model described what was lost:

I've been in practice 26 years. I've had two MAs, one for, like, 20 years and one for 16 years. ... You're like hand and glove. You just know exactly what each other is thinking. So that was really hard for me to be able to give that up [when we moved to a shared-MA model].

—primary care physician

Quantitative Findings

Among physicians responding to our survey, three in four reported having adequate numbers of support staff. The median respondent spent 95 percent of his or her work time in clinical activities, with one exclusive and ten shared allied health professionals. See Table 12.1.

Consistent with interviewee reports, analysis of survey data showed that having support staff members who were stable over time (i.e., with low turnover) was a statistically significant predictor of better overall professional satisfaction among physicians. There were also nonsignificant trends suggesting that greater shares of nonclinical time at work (devoted to management, teaching, research, or other activities) were associated with better satisfaction. In con-

Table 12.1
Responses to Survey Questions About Work Content and Support Staff

Item	Percentage	Median	Interquartile Range
Responding "Agree" or "Strongly agree" to the following:			
"I have enough support staff"	73		
Reporting the following:			
Share of work time that is nonclinical (%)		5	0–14
Number of exclusive allied health professionals (count per physician)		1	1–3
Number of shared allied health professionals (count per physician)		10	6–17

trast, the numbers of exclusive and shared allied health professionals were not associated with satisfaction in our sample. See Figure 12.1.

Comparison Between Current Findings and Previously Published Research

Our qualitative findings regarding work content and allocation of tasks among allied health professionals support staff are similar to those described in a recent study of high-performing primary care practices, which suggested that expanded roles for allied health professionals and support staff could address physician frustration and burnout (Sinsky et al., 2013).

We did not identify previous quantitative studies that assessed how specific tasks affected physician satisfaction. While questions pertaining to the burden of paperwork and the amount of administrative work required were included in the Physician Worklife Study as part of the "administration" facet of work, neither of these components was assessed independently in the study to determine its association with physician satisfaction (Wetterneck et al., 2002).

Figure 12.1
Adjusted Associations Between Measures of Work Content, Support, and Overall Professional Satisfaction

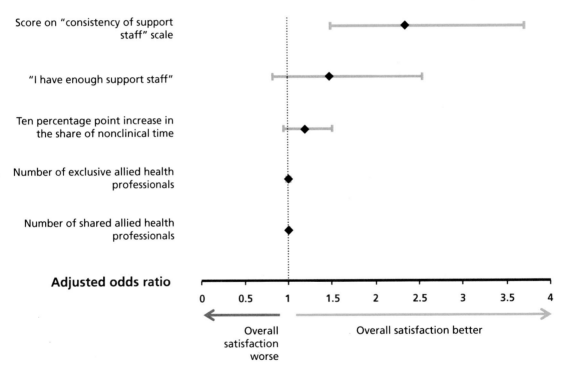

NOTES: Each estimate represents the effect of agreeing or strongly agreeing with the corresponding statement or a one-point increase in the corresponding continuous score. Effects are adjusted for practice size, specialty, and ownership, as well as for individually reported patient medical and social complexity and individual response tendency. 95-percent confidence intervals account for clustering of observations within practices. Statistically significant associations are highlighted by the use of colored confidence intervals: red for factors associated with worse satisfaction and green for factors associated with better satisfaction.
RAND *RR439-12.1*

CHAPTER THIRTEEN

Payment, Income, and Practice Finances

Overview of Findings

Although few physicians reported dissatisfaction with their current levels of income, physician income was an important contributor to satisfaction in the following ways:

- **Income stability.** Physicians reported that having a stable income was an important contributor to overall professional satisfaction, and some described taking steps to preserve their incomes when pay rates decreased (or other changes threatened to reduce income).
- **Income fairness.** Payment arrangements that were perceived as fair, transparent, and aligned with good patient care enhanced professional satisfaction. When practices changed their internal payment arrangements, clear and logical explanations for these changes were described as being important to preserving a sense of fairness.
- **Payment reform in the broader health care system.** Interviewees from practices of all specialties expressed a sense that relative incomes would shift, with primary care gaining and some subspecialties potentially losing income. This was a source of concern for some subspecialist physicians and for practices that had invested heavily in subspecialty care.

In addition, worries about practice financial sustainability, when present, were described as a source of dissatisfaction. For some physicians, working in practices in which they did not have an ownership interest (e.g., working for a hospital-owned practice) alleviated the stress associated with ownership.

In quantitative analyses of physician survey responses, we found that physicians in the highest quintiles of income and effective wage (annual income divided by annual hours worked) were significantly more likely to report overall professional satisfaction than those in the lowest quintiles. This finding contrasted with the interviews, either because interviewees may have given socially desirable responses (i.e., they may have downplayed the influence of overall income on professional satisfaction) or because those who earned higher incomes also found them to be fairer. Better overall satisfaction was associated significantly with greater perceived income fairness, positive perceived impact of individuals' clinical activities on practice finances, and satisfaction with income.

Qualitative Findings

Stability of Income

In our interviews, few physicians reported income level as a driver of satisfaction, and many described choosing not to maximize their incomes (e.g., by switching to another, higher-paying practice). However, physicians in a range of specialties commonly reported that having a stable, predictable income was important to professional satisfaction. Physicians who were earlier in their careers and facing significant financial commitments expressed this sentiment most clearly:

> Everyone would like to make a little bit more, but … nobody is leaving [the practice], … and it's no secret that you could make more working for one of the big HMOs. I mean, right now they're giving out huge signing bonuses which are really hard for us to compete with, but nobody's leaving. So, [income is] something that we'd all like to improve upon, but not to the point where we're willing to jump ship at all. … You know, some of us tend to be more nervous … those of us who are still paying off the mortgage and trying to put money in the kids' college accounts.
>
> —primary care physician

Some practice managers recognized the importance of income stability and sought to maintain competitive incomes for their physicians during periods of transition between payment models. One manager whose practice was transitioning from fee-for-service to value-based payment (via risk contracts with payers) explained:

> If you can figure out how to pay doctors a market-based salary while changing what they're doing, and it feels safe to them, then they are going to be the crucial movers to value. … We put a floor in on our physician salary such that their income with all this investment would not drop below a certain level. … We literally borrowed the money to get a three-year floor on physician salary so that, as we are [changing payment models], the hospitals couldn't come in and start picking off our doctors.
>
> —manager of a multispecialty practice

Fairness of Income

Across a range of specialties and practice models, physicians reported that earning an income that they perceived as fair was an important contributor to overall professional satisfaction.

Fairness as Transparency

While fairness could be judged in a variety of ways, physicians reported greater satisfaction when the methods for determining income were transparent, well understood, and equally applied within the practice:

> In the [obstetrics and gynecology] world, it takes nine months to actually get paid, because we get new patients, but we don't bill until after they deliver. And so the [obstetricians] had a two-year guaranteed salary, but then you become … production-based. But it's also very fair. [Our practice] is very, very open. … Like when we have our department meetings, and we do our compensation resets, we know how much everybody in our department makes

... because it's not hidden, we know: The harder you work, you know how much you'll get paid.

—obstetrician/gynecologist

Transparent incomes within a practice could also facilitate physician participation in new initiatives, especially when leaders' incomes were subject to the same level of transparency as full-time clinicians. The following leader of a corporate-owned practice described how such transparency could foster a greater sense of "ownership" and job satisfaction within the practice:

They see their [relative value units], they see their visits, and they see what they're making. Everybody knows in this practice what I'm making. In fact, they know what they're paying me as an administrative fee versus what I'm generating from the practice, and I know what so-and-so down the hall is doing. And we don't have to say anything; we just pass it out. ... And I tell them, I say, "Look, it's incumbent upon me to show that you're getting value from what you're paying me. You're not just paying me a salary because I'm wonderful, or I got appointed to this position. I earn this for you, and I want you to feel that way. And if I am not demonstrating to you that I am worth this stipend, you tell me, and either I gear up and do it, or you stop [paying me]." ... And [with this approach] you then get engagement, you get job satisfaction, you decrease burnout, all those things that come from feeling disenfranchised. So, at this practice, when I came on board as medical director, I said the first thing is, "I want everybody to feel like they own it." I want staff to feel that they own [the practice], that they're onboard, and that we are cohesive. And we're going to be transparent.

—primary care physician, medical director

Fairness as Good Explanations for Payment Changes

In general, physicians were willing to accept cuts to their own incomes as fair, as long as the cuts applied equally to all members of the practice and had a clear explanation. As one physician explained:

[Payment change] might be bad for everybody. It might be good for everybody. But as long as we know if it is fair, it's done this way, and you give us an explanation, [we can accept it]. For example, I think three or four years ago we used to get paid the same amount of money for all patients [regardless of payer]. [Then the practice] decided that we are not going to be able to do this for the people who have Medicaid, because Medicaid really does not pay very well. So they came across the system and they say, "We cannot do this anymore, it applies to all the system, this is how much we're going to reduce a payment for Medicaid, because we don't get reimbursed well for Medicaid." So it was hard to swallow, because it's a pay cut. ... But at the end of the day, they have a good explanation. It is systemwide. They're not singling out one group in one location saying, "We're going to do this to you."

—hematologist/oncologist

On the other hand, physicians were less tolerant of income reductions that were perceived as resulting from poor business decisions. Lower effective wages contributed to the following physician's decision to leave her previous practice:

My [previous practice] was having a hard time. They were trying to expand, and they had added on high-priced specialists and were building a sleep clinic and this and that. But the bottom line was that financially they ran into trouble, and they were having to have their physicians just work harder and harder for less and less. So they were basically on the verge of going under. ... I was making less and less, and seeing more and more patients, and being very harried.

—primary care physician

Fairness as Alignment Between Income and Good Patient Care

For some physicians, alignment between income and good care was a key factor in judging the fairness of their income. One physician who had transitioned from a prior position, in which his financial incentives were not aligned to good care, to a new position, in which his incentives were better aligned, explained:

[The largest local health plan] decided to start these quality report things. ... So, [in my old practice] I would get these reports every year, [which said]: "Look at you. Your patient satisfaction [is] off the chart. Quality metrics, you know, you're meeting it. And you're really low-cost." And I said: ... "You're getting out of me great value, and yet I don't get anything back from you. ... Do you see the irony in this? I'm killing myself and doing everything up front and taking care of my patients ... so why do I get paid the same flat rate as Joe Schmoe across the street who's a terrible doctor, costs you a lot of money, his outcomes are bad, he refers everything out, doesn't handle anything? ... Why should he and I receive the same [payment rates]?" ... So here [in my current practice], I get rewarded. If I came to do a good job, if I'm accessible to my patients, I get my good Press Ganey scores, if my access is good, if my quality metrics are good, I actually get rewarded. I like that. ... There's an alignment with my work and being compensated. And so, on the answer to the question, "Are you fairly compensated for what you do?" I strongly agree.

—primary care physician

On the other hand, financial incentives to provide better care could produce dissatisfaction when physicians lacked the resources and guidance to improve. For example, one practice leader explained how the practice had learned from a prior misstep in this regard:

We set [patient satisfaction] as a goal. However, we didn't necessarily align resources with helping physicians to be able to achieve those goals. There was a lot of dissatisfaction with that. We've sort of taken a restart. ... We've taken a different approach, saying, "Okay, how do we provide resources to help the physicians to improve?" ... [We are] getting out and explaining to folks why this is important and providing tools for them to be able to enhance their performance ... and develop a culture of service from the ground up.

—leader of a multispecialty practice

Payment Reform

Interviewees from practices of all specialties expressed a sense that relative incomes would shift, with primary care gaining and physicians in some subspecialties potentially losing income. This was a source of concern for some single-subspecialty practices and for multispecialty practices that had invested heavily in subspecialty care:

The fact that we've got a lot of specialty care within the organization, I think, is going to make it tougher and tougher over time. ... [Because of payment reform,] we do have to make that decision about where we're heading with specialty care, where we're heading with primary care, and how those two kind of meet, because as far as I can tell, it's good news for primary care, because they might have been downtrodden for too long and not appreciated, but that curve is going up. The specialty curve is heading down. So, we need to find a way to maintain an organizational success with that model, because we've been very specialty-driven over the years. And you'll continue to need [specialty care], but at what level?

—administrator of a multispecialty practice

As I look across the benchmarking metrics of different types of doctors, the specialties and the primary care doctors … the income differential is so vast that I don't believe that it's sustainable. You know something is gonna have to evolve in that respect. Hopefully, the primary care doctors' incomes go up and the specialists' incomes are not adversely affected downward. Whether that is the case or not is impossible to predict. But certainly, I think you have to expect that there's gonna be some type of material, substantial change in the incomes that physicians receive for the services they provide to different patients in different specialties in our delivery system.

—manager of a surgical subspecialty practice

Concerns About Practice Financial Sustainability

Worries about practice financial sustainability, when present, were described as a source of dissatisfaction. For some physicians, working in practices in which they did not have an ownership interest (e.g., working for a hospital-owned practice) alleviated the financial stress associated with ownership. As one practice administrator explained, the loss of autonomy when a partnership practice was sold to a hospital was counterbalanced by higher incomes and decoupling of practice and personal finances:

Most of [the physicians in the practice] now are making more money than they've ever made in their life, but they're not 100 percent in charge any more, you know, so I think that there's some [downside]. … But, at the same time, … the former owners of this group … will tell that they sleep much better at night knowing that they are not signed onto some big note for debt.

—practice administrator

Quantitative Findings

Approximately 85 percent of survey respondents reported their earnings from clinical activities in the prior year, and nearly all reported their work hours. To calculate each physician's "effective wage," we divided his or her reported income by the total number of hours worked in the prior year. Incomes and effective wages varied widely, as shown in Table 13.1.

Among physicians responding to our survey, most agreed that their total compensation packages were fair and were satisfied with their benefits. Factors reflecting personal productivity and practice overall financial performance had the greatest influence on personal income. See Table 13.2.

Table 13.1
Reported Earnings Among Survey Respondents

	Quintile	Amount
Effective wage ($ per hour)	5 (highest)	158 or more
	4	115–157
	3	92–114
	2	73–91
	1 (lowest)	72 or less
Income ($ per year)	5 (highest)	350,001 or more
	4	250,001–350,000
	3	200,001–250,000
	2	160,001–200,000
	1 (lowest)	160,000 or less

Table 13.2
Responses to Survey Questions About Payment, Income, and Practice Finances

Category and Item	Percentage
Fairness and satisfaction with compensation (responding "Agree" or "Strongly agree")	
"My total compensation package is fair"	71
"I am not well compensated given my training and experience"	22
"I am not well compensated compared to physicians in other specialties"	44
"I am not well compensated compared to other physicians in my practice"	11
"I regularly receive information about the practices overall financial position"	76
"I receive information about how my own clinical activities impact practice finances"	56
"The methods used to calculate my financial impact on the practice are fair"	57
"I am told that my clinical activities have a positive impact on practice finances"	56
"I am told that on the balance, my clinical activities are a net financial loss to the practice"	8
"I am satisfied with the benefits (e.g., health insurance) I receive in my current job"	79
Importance of the following factors in determining compensation (responding Very or Moderately Important)	
Factors reflecting your own productivity	81
The overall financial performance of the practice	71
Results of satisfaction surveys completed by your patients	27
Specific measures of quality of care such as rates of preventive care services for your patients	32
Results of practice profiling (i.e., comparing your pattern of using medical resources with that of other physicians)	19

In quantitative analyses of physician survey responses, we found that physicians in the highest quintiles of income and effective wage were significantly more likely to report overall professional satisfaction than those in the lowest quintiles. This finding contrasted with the interviews, in which income levels were not identified as major contributors to satisfaction. This disagreement between qualitative and quantitative findings has at least two potential explanations. First, interviewees may have given socially desirable responses by downplaying the influence of overall income on their professional satisfaction. Second, those who earned higher incomes may have also found them to be fairer. See Figure 13.1.

Congruent with interview findings, physicians were more likely to be satisfied when they perceived their compensation as fair, when they received feedback indicating that their own clinical activities had a positive impact on practice finances, and when they were satisfied with their overall level of compensation. Better overall satisfaction also was associated significantly with satisfaction with benefits—a topic not probed in the interviews. See Figure 13.2.

Figure 13.1
Adjusted Associations Between Measures of Income and Overall Professional Satisfaction

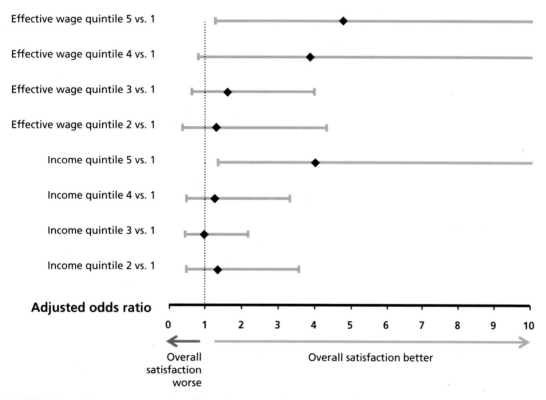

NOTES: Each estimate represents the effect of reporting the corresponding category of effective wage (income divided by total hours worked per year) or income in the prior year. For wages and income, quintile 5 is the highest, and quintile 1 is the lowest. Odds ratios are adjusted for practice size, specialty, and ownership, as well as for individual seniority (years in practice) and response tendency. 95-percent confidence intervals account for clustering of observations within practices. Statistically significant associations are highlighted by the use of colored confidence intervals: red for factors associated with worse satisfaction and green for factors associated with better satisfaction.
RAND *RR439-13.1*

Figure 13.2
Adjusted Associations Between Perceptions of Income, Personal Impact on Practice Finances, and Overall Professional Satisfaction

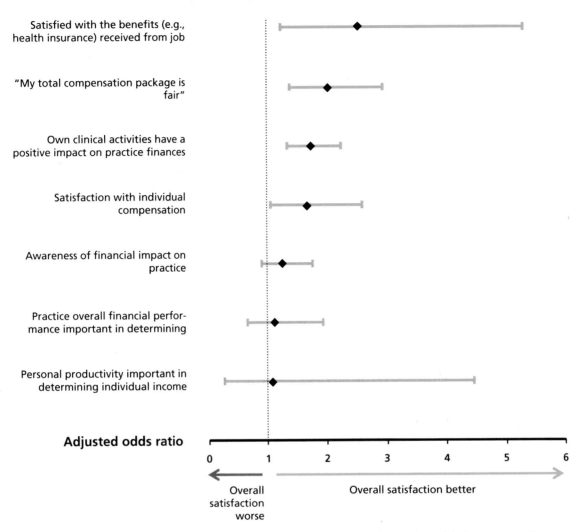

NOTES: Each estimate represents the effect of reporting agreeing or strongly agreeing with the corresponding statement or a one-point increase in the corresponding continuous score. Effects are adjusted for practice size, specialty, and ownership, as well as for individual seniority (years in practice) and response tendency. 95-percent confidence intervals account for clustering of observations within practices. Statistically significant associations are highlighted by the use of colored confidence intervals: red for factors associated with worse satisfaction or green for factors associated with better satisfaction.
RAND *RR439-13.2*

Comparison Between Current Findings and Previously Published Research

Similar to our findings, prior research in multiple practice settings has found that physician perception of earning a "fair" income is a strong predictor of overall satisfaction (Movassaghi and Kindig, 1989; Linn et al., 1986; Warren, Weitz and Kulis, 1998). Some previous research has also found higher incomes associated with greater professional satisfaction (Boukus, Cassil and O'Malley, 2009; Leigh, Tancredi and Kravitz, 2009; Cydulka and Korte, 2008; Lewis et al., 1993a), although several studies based on data from the Community Tracking Study/

Health Tracking Physician Survey indicated a slight drop in satisfaction among those in the highest income brackets—contrary to findings within our study sample (Chen et al., 2012; Leigh et al., 2002; Stoddard et al., 2001).

CHAPTER FOURTEEN

Regulatory and Professional Liability Concerns

Overview of Findings

Physicians and practice managers described externally imposed rules and regulations under which they operated as having predominantly negative effects on professional satisfaction. Among these, meaningful-use rules stood out as having the greatest effect on professional satisfaction at the time of this study. While physicians agreed generally with the intent of meaningful-use rules, they expressed frustration with the time and documentation burdens these rules imposed—especially when they believed they were being asked to generate new documentation of activities that they had already performed.

The prominence of meaningful-use regulations in our interviews may reflect the particular timing of this study, which was conducted while many practices were adopting or changing their EHRs. A similar study conducted a few years earlier or later would probably identify other specific regulations as especially influential for professional satisfaction. However, as interviewees described, the cumulative effect of a large number of rules and regulations (from a wide variety of sources, not limited to government) on professional satisfaction may be a more long-standing finding.

Professional liability concerns were not prominent contributors to dissatisfaction among the practices we sampled. As our interviews revealed, recent reforms of professional liability laws may have contributed to this finding. Consistent with interview findings, analysis of survey data did not reveal associations between overall professional satisfaction and the professional liability issues we investigated.

Qualitative Findings

Cumulative Effect of Many Rules and Regulations: Frustration and Burnout

Physicians of all specialties reported feeling overwhelmed by the cumulative effect of rules and regulations on their ability to deliver patient care or run a practice. These frustrations were present in all practice models, but physicians in small and medium-sized practices expressed these frustrations most strongly. Other than meaningful use, which is detailed in the next section, no single rule or set of regulations stood out as being especially burdensome. Instead, informants described the sheer volume of regulations as problematic, either because of the resulting expenses for the practice or because of a sense of "attack":

> I think the biggest challenge is still regulation over health care—governmental regulation, insurance company regulation, all the different deals of just what we have to do. ...

For total joint [replacements], the government now has five criteria to jump through. ... Meaningful Use One, [Physician Quality Reporting System] data, Meaningful Use Two, all these different things are just sapping our strength. ... [And] we're going to need more people, because of the regulations, to do the same job.

—orthopedic surgeon

I think that the amount of work, the amount of complicated red tape, et cetera, for the level of reimbursement, one curve is going up, the other curve is going down, and it really is changing the face of what a physician is. ... And it's not just from the government, it's from malpractice; at every single turn, you feel [an] attack or constraint or manipulation or mandate. ... There are times when you wonder: Do people really care about physicians? Do they have anything good to feel or say or do with them? ... It's a profession that's gone under a lot of attack, that perhaps parts of it were necessary, and there were some people that needed to be different. But just like so many changes, the size of it ends up being bigger than the need.

—general surgeon

The complexity of payment rules, especially for new types of fee-for-service payment, has been difficult for some physicians:

Medicare ... has the annual wellness visit that they pay for. But ... it's just a nightmare, the rules of whether you can do it. There's three different levels of it: On this [level] you can do X, and this [other] one you can't do that, and this [third] one you can only do these five things—It's ridiculous. I mean, it probably took us a year and a half to get it straight, and still there's a lot of confusion. ... So this year, it was the transitional care management. So this is a fee: Patient comes out of hospital; you can charge it one time in a month. You couldn't tell if it was separate from a visit or in addition to a visit. How much was it going to pay? And then we got them all denied. Well, it turns out you have to bill it on the day that is 30 days from the date of discharge. [The instructions] never said that. But so basically we turned in like 15 of them in the first two months and they were all denied. ... No wonder doctors don't embrace some of these [new payment models]. ... They're making it way too complex for the average primary care doctor to grasp. Put it in writing. Here are the ten rules. I can follow the ten rules. But usually what happens is I have to read in about ten different places to figure out why we did not get paid.

—primary care physician

Meaningful-Use Requirements Are Perceived as Good for Patient Care but Are Time Consuming and Frustrating for Some Physicians

Among the regulations affecting professional satisfaction, meaningful-use rules were the specific rules most commonly and prominently mentioned by interviewees. In general, physicians and practice managers believed that meaningful-use rules encouraged better patient care. At the same time, however, these rules significantly increased the time and staffing needed to deliver patient care:

So, when we first transitioned over [to an EHR], it definitely increased time it took for charting, ... And then now with the meaningful-use stuff, that just added that many more clicks and things that you have to do. ... So, all of those things just keep adding time that we didn't necessarily have to begin with. Each patient visit is taking much, much longer, including staff stuff because [meaningful use] added stuff they had to do. ... [But] you know, I would say although it does add time, and it's, you know, a bit of a painful thing, those changes that have been made do make things better. ... Reviewing the medications, which is part of the meaningful use; I mean our med list used to ... just go on forever with all these antibiotics that were never discontinued. And so, now people having to clean that up, it makes for a much better medical record.

—pediatrician

Some physicians who already had EHRs described the primary effect of "meaningful use" as increased documentation. To the extent that meaningful use represented an exercise in documentation rather than a beneficial change in patient care, physicians and practice managers found the new rules frustrating:

It's frustrating from my standpoint that [with] "meaningful use" ... we have all of these rules that we have to follow now. For example, we have been counseling on diet, exercise, [body mass index], all of these things for years. ... So we've been doing the work, but unless we change the way we state things and the way we're coding, we don't get credit for it. It's been frustrating trying to figure out how [to] do that but not lose efficiency.

—primary care physician

[The EHR] supersedes everything by far. "Meaningful use," you know, that's coming down the pike and the changes [are] huge. And it just ... it's more and more and more and more. You know, every meeting it's, like, there's new things added to the list ... and some of it's really good. But a lot of it is stuff we already do because it's good patient care, but now we have to figure out how to do it so that they can count it and get credit for it—which is really frustrating. That's not why I went to medical school. ... I just want to take care of the patient.

—physician manager of a multispecialty practice

Improvements in the Professional Liability Environment Contributed to Better Professional Satisfaction

In the states included in our study, some of which had adopted professional liability reforms, physicians described their new professional liability environments as enhancing their professional satisfaction:

[Professional liability reform] has been awesome. ... The lawyers were like a feeding frenzy. And right before they changed the law, they had a little feeding frenzy where they said, "If you think a doctor did you wrong, call us and we'll sue them"—because they knew all those huge judgments were going to go away. ... I think there's doctors that probably need to be sued. Bad things happen. You cut off somebody's leg that's the wrong leg—those people need to be sued. But there were a lot of nonsense lawsuits out there, and we saw those [decrease]. My malpractice insurance is less now than it was when I started.

—primary care physician

Among the practices that we visited, professional liability concerns were described as relatively minor stressors. As one surgeon described, alternative mechanisms for compensating patients were a source of comfort:

I think [professional liability] is always on your mind, but I don't think it's terrible. I think we do have fairly good tort laws here that protect us, and ... our insurance is pretty good about, you know, getting rid of the frivolous suit right from the beginning, basically just kind of shooing them away. ... We also have, within our insurance provider, a really good program called "Three Rs," where basically if an unanticipated outcome occurs, you can contact [the insurer], and they will offer assistance to the patient as far as managing lost wages and unforeseen medical expenses, unforeseen expenses at home. ... It's really just designed to kind of ease some of [those expenses] and, hopefully, let the patient know that we do care about them and that we are concerned about the fact that [their outcome] wasn't anticipated. It doesn't preclude them from filing a suit; however, ... it does seem to have reduced the suits significantly.

—general surgeon

Quantitative Findings

Our survey assessed physician respondents' experiences with professional liability (malpractice) lawsuits and asked how the practice handled such lawsuits. Fewer than one in five physicians responding to our survey had personal experience as a professional liability defendant while working at his or her current practice. Consistent with this finding, the majority of survey respondents did not know how the interests of individual physicians would be balanced with those of the practice in the event of a lawsuit. Our survey did not assess physicians' experiences with regulations affecting their practices. See Table 14.1.

In our sample, there were no statistically significant relationships between experiences with professional liability lawsuits or the balance of interests in the defense of such lawsuits and professional satisfaction. See Figure 14.1.

Comparison Between Current Findings and Previously Published Research

Evidence on how legal and regulatory requirements are affecting physician satisfaction was sparse in existing literature. One study utilizing data from the Physician Worklife Study reported that the "hassle factor" stemming from economic and regulatory forces external to the practice organization (e.g., insurance authorizations and gatekeeping requirements) was significantly and negatively correlated with satisfaction (Konrad et al., 1999). To our knowledge, the effects of more recent requirements, such as "meaningful use," on physician satisfaction have not yet been reported in previously published literature.

Table 14.1
Responses to Survey Questions About Professional Liability

Item	Percentage
"Have you ever been the defendant in a professional liability (malpractice) lawsuit while working at this practice?"	
Yes	17
No	83
"When there is a professional liability (malpractice) lawsuit against a doctor in this practice, can the doctor choose his or her legal representation?"	
Yes, the doctor chooses	16
No, the practice chooses	27
Don't know	57
"When there is a professional liability (malpractice) lawsuit against a doctor in this practice, which of the following most accurately describes the defense of the doctor?"	
The priority will be to defend the doctor, even if this might be more expensive for the practice	23
The defense will balance the needs of the doctor and the needs of the practice	15
The defense will seek to settle the suit quickly, even if this may result in a negative notation in the doctor's personal record	3
Don't know	59

Figure 14.1
Adjusted Associations Between Professional Liability Concerns and Overall Professional Satisfaction

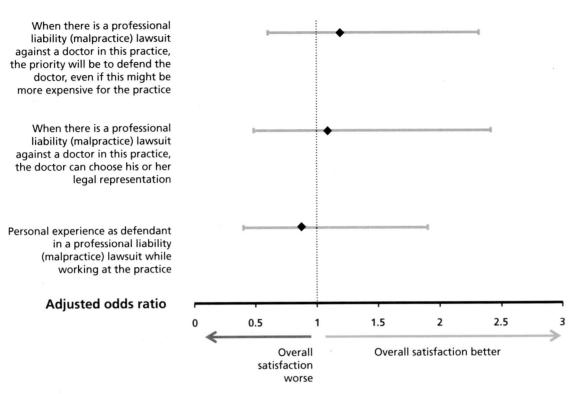

NOTES: Each estimate represents the effect of reporting the corresponding category. Odds ratios are adjusted for practice size, specialty, and ownership, as well as for individual seniority (years in practice) and response tendency. 95-percent confidence intervals account for clustering of observations within practices. Statistically significant associations are highlighted by the use of colored confidence intervals: red for factors associated with worse satisfaction and green for factors associated with better satisfaction.

RAND *RR439-14.1*

CHAPTER FIFTEEN

Health Reform

Overview of Findings

Our study did not identify health reform as a prominent contributor to overall physician professional satisfaction, either positively or negatively. In general, physicians and administrators expressed uncertainty about how various aspects of health reform (including but not limited to those contained in the Affordable Care Act) would affect physician satisfaction and practice financial sustainability. In response to this uncertainty, several practices sought economic security by increasing in size or becoming affiliated with hospitals and large delivery systems. Leaders of smaller, independent practices that did not initiate such growth or affiliation described feeling pressure to join larger systems, sensing that it would become more difficult in the future to remain independent from these systems as a consequence of health reform.

In addition to this general uncertainty, interviewees described some specific concerns. First, the transition from one payment model (fee-for-service) to a new payment model (e.g., shared savings or capitation) would be complicated, with physicians receiving mixed incentives from different payers. Second, primary care physicians generally expressed support for the PCMH model. However, some in our sample were dissatisfied by increased paperwork, and others expressed concern about whether delegating too much responsibility to other types of providers and staff could compromise the quality of care.

In quantitative analyses, there were no statistically significant associations between practice participation in the new payment or delivery models we investigated (shared savings, episode-based payment, ACOs, PCMHs) and overall physician professional satisfaction. This finding is concordant with the qualitative finding that health reform had low prominence among the factors affecting physician professional satisfaction, but it could also be a consequence of limited sample size (i.e., with 30 practices in the study, only a small number participated in any given new payment or delivery model).

Qualitative Findings

Uncertainty About the Effects of Health Reform as Leading to Consolidation

Overall, respondents in our study expressed uncertainty over the effects of health reform more broadly (and the Affordable Care Act specifically) on their practices and on themselves as individuals. At the same time, multiple practices in our sample had made "educated guesses" as to the direction and effects of reform, and some had taken steps to maintain their local market positions, most commonly by becoming larger themselves or by joining larger delivery systems.

The following practice chief executive officer described how becoming part of a larger system was expected to improve the practice's stability:

> If you would have said to me five years ago that I would be in an integration package with [our hospital], I would have said, "There is no way in hell I would be in this package." [Yet] here I am. … Our sole reason for being part of the [hospital] health system is security— actually, several sole reasons, but [mainly] security. But we believe that it's going to be a single payer model … somewhere in the future. And you have to be closely aligned with a hospital system in a positive way in order for anybody to survive. … And we believe that market share is going to be based on not volume of procedures, but on [number of patients]. So we want to make our future so that we can have the biggest number of patients come to [our practice] so that our reimbursement, which will be by patient, is going to be at a high level.
>
> —CEO of a medical subspecialty practice

An administrator of a surgical practice expressed similar sentiments:

> I think the biggest thing right now is just all the regulations and Obamacare and just the uncertainty of what's coming down the pike. Nobody knows, everybody tries to speculate, they're trying to position themselves so that they don't all of a sudden fall behind or out of the picture completely. … I think our doctors feel being a large entity, that [practice financial sustainability problems] might not happen to them as easily as it could happen to a one- or two-doctor practice.
>
> —administrator of a surgical practice

Practice leaders who saw full capitation as a future possible payment model viewed sharing financial risk with hospitals as a way to better mitigate the high costs of hospitalization. This constituted another reason to affiliate with hospitals:

> In the long term, you hope that you can partner with a payer [so that] you're really getting paid more … like a managed care contract, where they're going to pay you so much per month [per patient]. … We feel like we're in a position that we could take on a lot more risk down the road, but you [have] to make sure that your alliance with the hospital … is in place, because all it takes is a couple of trips over there [by patients], and your margin gets eroded.
>
> —CEO of a multispecialty practice

Leaders of some independent practices that were not actively seeking to affiliate with larger systems described feeling pressure to join larger systems, sensing that it would become more difficult in the future to remain independent from these systems as a consequence of health reform. In some cases, this pressure came from large local delivery systems directly, as the following leader of a primary care practice described:

> In the past it was very easy [to remain independent]. … Just a couple weeks ago, [a large local delivery system] sort of made the statement, "We're going to build something right next door, or let us acquire you." [We said:] "Well, no, we're not going to let you acquire us." So, okay, and now next week later I get a call: "We've rethought this. Can we rent some

space from you and put our specialists in your building?" And so I think they're trying to figure out how they're going to work, too. In the end, the system is forcing, I think, some alignments. And at some point we're going to have to choose allegiances, which is unfortunate. I think it's worked well for our patients to have [multiple options for referrals to subspecialty care], and they're going to lose that now. ... Because of the way the payment systems are moving, we're going to have to be with one system or another. ... To manage risk now, you have to have a larger pool to be able to get the dollars in, and we won't have that larger pool. So, we'll have to be part of someone else's pool.

—primary care physician

Transitions from One Payment Model to Another

Physicians and leaders in a variety of practice models believed that fee-for-service payment would be replaced by shared savings, bundled payment, or other value-based models of payment. Some expressed concerns about how to transition smoothly from one payment system to another. As one physician described, changes in payment models would necessitate changes in the allocation of tasks among a team of caregivers, but changing to team-based care too quickly, before fundamental payment changes took hold, would jeopardize the practice's financial sustainability:

> I think the biggest challenge is going to be to splice together the reimbursement that's based on widgets—how many patients you see in a day determines how much you get paid—and transitioning that payment and reimbursement model into what's coming. ... The new model is [that] the provider shouldn't be doing that work; somebody who doesn't cost as much should be doing that work, and somebody [who] probably could do better than the provider should be doing that work. ... We're in between those two practice models now. And that's really hard, because if we transition too much to give away work to those who should be doing it, then our income goes way down, because ... that's not how we're getting paid yet.

—primary care physician

A number of subspecialists foresaw similar challenges, including how to pay physicians within a subspecialty practice, as one orthopedic surgeon described:

> Fee for services is gonna be gone, it's just a matter of when. ... An orthopedic surgeon will be paid on bundled payment, I think, eventually. And so we need to somehow be able to bridge the gap, so to speak, which is going to be difficult particularly with physician compensation. How do I still have one foot still in the fee-for-service world ... for the patients that do see us [under] fee-for-service until they're completely in ACO, and then how do I pay physicians that are being bundled for their procedures?

—orthopedic surgeon

Medical Homes

Most primary care practices in our sample had chosen to become "medical homes" (also known as patient-centered medical homes) and were either in the process of applying for medical home recognition (from the National Committee for Quality Assurance and other bodies) or had already received such recognition. Some practices had participated in early medical home pilots; interviewees from these practices reported that the paperwork involved in pilot participation and medical home recognition was a significant burden. However, some participants also reported that becoming a medical home had resulted in a more efficient delegation of work from physicians to other team members. As one pilot participant described:

> In that pilot, we had to go through the process of becoming patient-centered medical home certified. … There were a lot of changes that had to be made, and we had to document a lot of stuff. We had to produce a lot of information. It was very painful, and at the time, I kind of resented that. … But I will tell you that, on the other side of that doorway, it's been really good. I mean, it's been a really very positive thing; whether we were paid for it or not, it's been a really positive thing for our practice. I think a lot of people look at patient-centered medical home as, "It's just a ticket I have to get punched so that I can get paid for this or paid for that." And [they're] really not seeing that it really is a real change in how you practice. In the past, I felt from my training that I had to do it all. And I think one of the messages that came down to me [from the pilot was that] I needed to push out a lot of the stuff that I was doing to other people. Obviously they need to be trained. I need to trust them. There needs to be accountability. But that I don't have to do [everything]. … So when I have a patient come in, the nurse talks to them about their mammogram and gives them their tetanus booster. The nurse makes sure that they're set up for X, Y, and Z. So, then, I can sit down and talk to them about [why their] diabetes isn't under control. So I think that's a big change.
>
> —primary care physician, leader of a small practice

However, some physicians voiced concern about turning over important aspects of care to other types of providers and staff. To the extent that a medical home model may give physicians a more managerial role, with less direct contact with their patients, the following physician worried about unintended effects on the quality of care, especially for complex patients:

> I'm concerned a little bit about seeing increasing divestment of primary care to midlevel practitioners, who I think do a great job for many problems using [a] kind of a protocol-driven way of thinking about those problems. And I realize the patients are often satisfied and happy with the care that they're given. I still am concerned because—perhaps more in the nursing home population where I see a lot of nuances and outliers as far as problems—that sometimes things don't get fully addressed. And there is an element of needing to have somebody with a bit more experience, at some point, in taking care of frail and complicated patients—[a provider] who may know, just from training experience, those nuances in a little more detail. … But increasingly we're being asked, as physicians, to provide more of a supervisory role and not necessarily … having as much hands-on or eyes-on experience with patients. And so that's a concern that I have for the future with the whole area of group care and the patient-centered [medical] home. … I'm uncomfortable sometimes thinking about frail elderly patients and not seeing them that often. I'm concerned about just signing off on someone else's work. … I'm not sure how far we can extend without starting to compromise the care that we would like to give and that people expect.
>
> —primary care physician

Quantitative Findings

Among the practices in the study, approximately one-half were participating in a new payment or delivery system model. See Table 15.1.

Analysis of physician survey responses revealed no significant relationships between practice engagement in new payment or delivery system models and overall professional satisfaction, a finding that seems congruent with the uncertainties expressed about how health reform will affect physician practices. The absence of observed quantitative associations may also stem from the earliness of these new payment models; when present, few practices had more than a year or two of experience with them. In addition, these null findings could be explained by limited power: For practice-level variables, such as participation in new payment or delivery models, statistical power is dependent on the number of practices. Therefore, a lack of association between the new payment and delivery models investigated and physician professional satisfaction would need to be confirmed in a larger sample before being considered "proof of no effect." See Figure 15.1.

Comparison Between Current Findings and Previously Published Research

We did not find strong qualitative or quantitative relationships between health reform and physician professional satisfaction, and the Affordable Care Act and associated models of care delivery (e.g., medical homes and ACOs) are too recent to have been extensively studied in the published literature.

However, existing evidence in potentially related areas, such as expansions in managed care and HMOs in the 1980s and 1990s, may allow useful comparison. In these older studies, managed care had mixed effects on physician satisfaction. Physicians in markets with larger proportions of managed care reported lower professional satisfaction in a variety of studies (Leigh, Tancredi and Kravitz, 2009; Landon et al., 2002; Buchbinder et al., 2001; Warren, Weitz and Kulis, 1998). This finding was especially pronounced among primary care physicians, who reported a significant decline in satisfaction due to managed care, while the effect among specialists was not significant (Landon, Reschovsky and Blumenthal, 2003).

Table 15.1
Responses to Practice Structural Questionnaire Items on Payment and Delivery Models

Payment or Delivery Model	Practices Participating in Model (all or part of practice)[a]
Accountable care organization (ACO)	15
Patient-centered medical home	15
Shared savings	14
Episode-based payment	6

[a] Out of 29 practices that completed the practice structural questionnaire.

Figure 15.1
Adjusted Associations Between Practice Participation in New Payment Models and Overall Professional Satisfaction

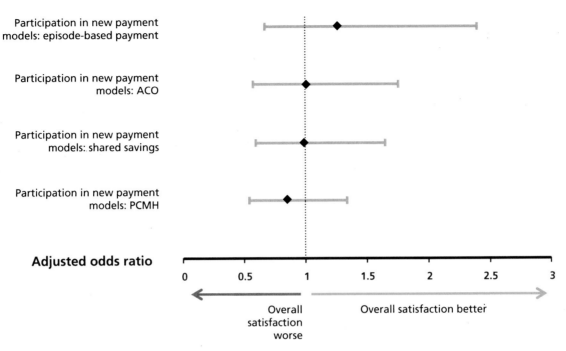

NOTES: Each estimate represents the effect of practice participation in the corresponding type of payment reform. Odds ratios are adjusted for practice size, specialty, and ownership, as well as for individual respondent seniority (number of years in practice) and response tendency. 95-percent confidence intervals account for clustering of observations within practices. Statistically significant associations are highlighted by the use of colored confidence intervals: red for factors associated with worse satisfaction and green for factors associated with better satisfaction.

RAND RR439-15.1

CHAPTER SIXTEEN

Conclusions

Most physicians included in this study were generally satisfied with their medical practices, similar to prior studies of overall physician professional satisfaction. However, a substantial minority of physicians report low professional satisfaction, and even those who are generally satisfied with their careers describe a range of specific factors that substantially frustrate, stress, or otherwise dissatisfy them. Many of these sources of dissatisfaction are remediable, and, importantly, many seem likely to detract from the quality and efficiency of patient care. Therefore, interventions to remediate the most troubling of these sources of dissatisfaction seem necessary and timely.

Our study found that physicians are more satisfied when they perceive that they are delivering high-quality care and meeting their patients' needs—and are dissatisfied when they perceive that the opposite is true. To the extent that physicians' perceptions about quality are correct, this finding suggests an additional way of thinking about the relationship between physician professional satisfaction and the quality of care that patients receive. Aside from viewing better patient care as a potential "downstream" benefit of better physician professional satisfaction, it may be useful to view physician dissatisfaction, when it is caused by perceived quality problems, as an indicator of potential delivery system dysfunction.

In this view, the critical step is to understand *why* some physicians report dissatisfaction with some aspects of their professional lives, even when overall satisfaction is high. Some obstacles to professional satisfaction may have limited direct relationships with the quality of care, but when dissatisfaction stems from factors that physicians perceive as compromising the quality of patient care, further investigation of these factors may help identify important opportunities to improve patient care.

Putting this point another way, the relationship between changes in professional satisfaction and changes in the quality and efficiency of patient care is likely to depend heavily on the exact reasons that professional satisfaction is changing. Without understanding these reasons, relationships between overall professional satisfaction and the quality of patient care will be difficult to interpret or predict in a useful way. For example, it seems possible to improve professional satisfaction without improving patient care (e.g., by giving physicians more time off, without taking steps to maintain patient access to care), and such an intervention would be unattractive to many stakeholders. However, the majority of sources of dissatisfaction identified in our study represent forms of delivery system dysfunction that many stakeholders would like to see solved: insufficient time per patient, EHRs with poor usability, regulations that require physicians to spend time on tasks that do not require their training, high turnover rates among allied health professionals and support staff, etc. Interventions that target these delivery system problems would be expected to improve professional satisfaction while, at the same time, enhancing patient care.

Our findings suggest several targets for interventions that, if successful, seem likely to benefit patients, physicians, and allied health professionals alike. We divide these into targets internal to physician practices and targets external to physician practices (including those that would involve many physician practices). Finally, we will discuss questions of public and private policy that will need to be answered to design successful interventions.

Improvement Targets: Internal to Physician Practices

Within practices, sources of low physician professional satisfaction may warrant systematic examination and interventions. Time pressure, lack of control over day-to-day decisions that affect patient care, and loss of collegiality are all causes of dissatisfaction that are within the purview of the practice to address. Interventions that can address the following sources of physician professional dissatisfaction seem most likely to improve patient care:

- **Time pressure detracting from the care experience.** Physicians in multiple specialties and all practice models included in this study described having insufficient time to deliver what they perceived as high-quality patient care. At the same time, however, many physicians—especially those without large numbers of dedicated allied health professionals and support staff—described spending a significant amount of time performing tasks that did not truly require a physician's training and that "crowd out" those that did. For example, such activities as filling out forms, typing and correcting automated transcriptions, dealing with onerous EHR order entry screens, and other "secretarial" duties were reported as occupying a significant share of physicians' time. While these are important activities and, in some cases, regulations or laws may mandate that a physician perform them, they are not truly activities in which physicians work to the "top of their licenses." Interventions that can reallocate these activities to other staff (or dispense with them altogether, when appropriate) may free physicians' time to devote to patient care tasks that truly require their training, thereby improving the quality of care, the patient care experience, and professional satisfaction. However, such practice transformations are likely to require resources, time, and an appropriate regulatory environment (i.e., one that does not force physicians to perform below-license tasks) to execute successfully.
- **Lack of a sense of control over day-to-day decisions affecting patient care.** We found that physicians who report greater control over the pace and content of their work and those who have a sense of ownership of and responsibility for their practices have better professional satisfaction than do those who report less control over day-to-day decisions affecting patient care. This finding appeared to be true irrespective of practice size but was related to whether individual physicians felt connected to the decisions that influence their practice environment. This sense of control could be weakened by a number of factors, including inadequate communication mechanisms within the practice, perceived obscurity or unfairness of within-practice payment mechanisms, and having to use unworkable EHRs. In addition, lack of clarity about the role of physicians in the leadership and management of hospital-based integrated systems was a new cause of anxiety. Policies and procedures that allow physicians to participate in practice management, in

both ownership and employed-physician practice environments, may improve physicians' sense of control over factors that directly affect their delivery of patient care.

- **Loss of collegiality and subsequent feelings of isolation.** A number of factors contributed to a diminished sense of connectedness among physicians, leading to feelings of isolation and having to "go it alone" (even within some medium and large practices). These factors included a loss of regular business meetings with other physicians in the practice (as a consequence of moving from physician-owned to hospital-owned practice models), less time spent with colleagues in the hospital setting (due to movement of procedures out of the institution and the advent of hospitalists), competitive relationships between practices, and ever-present time pressure, which left little time for social interaction during the workday. While some of these factors may be difficult to address without cooperation across practices, practices that do not already have regular business meetings could create other opportunities for physicians to communicate, share, and learn from one another in a face-to-face setting.

- **Stress due to change.** Even when change was desired, adopting new practice models, payment systems, and technologies was stressful for many physician practices. Insufficient organizational slack, frequently expressed as time pressure (e.g., a sensation of "running on a treadmill" just to finish each day's work), discouraged physicians from making changes that would ultimately improve their professional satisfaction. While some physicians we interviewed had developed innovative practice models or engaged in major workflow redesign efforts, most described greater risk aversion. A clear set of proven pathways to new practice models for physician practices in a variety of starting positions, coupled with resources to create organizational slack, could reduce the stresses of change.

Improvement Targets: External to Physician Practices

External to the individual practice, our study identified a number of larger health system issues. These targets included deficiencies in EHR technology, the cumulative burden of regulations, relationships between physicians and the hospitals and health systems that employ physicians, and physician payment policies.

- **Deficiencies in EHR technology.** While EHRs have many benefits for physicians, including the ability to remotely access patient information and the larger promise of improvements in the quality of care, numerous physicians reported problems with these systems that contributed to overall professional dissatisfaction. Across a wide range of EHR software products and practice models, physicians reported poor EHR usability, time-consuming data entry, interference with face-to-face patient care, degraded clinical documentation (as a consequence of template-based notes), and inefficient and less fulfilling work content. In addition, the inability to exchange health information between EHRs limited the ultimate effectiveness of these products.

  These findings suggest that the current state of EHR technology may be insufficient to deliver on the promise of EHRs. While there are some internal practice improvements that can be used, such as scribes, a larger system view is needed to improve the technology. Collaboration between EHR vendors, physician professional associations, hospitals, and other provider groups to improve the usability and interoperability of these products will be essential. In addition, federal EHR certification criteria should include, in some form, the notion that a minimum level of system usability will be necessary to have desired effects on the quality and efficiency of patient care. Our research found that physicians are optimistic about the future of EHR technology, but current inadequacies in the current (hopefully, transitional) state of EHRs must be addressed quickly.

- **The cumulative burden of regulations.** Physicians and practice managers described the externally imposed rules and regulations under which they operated as having predominantly negative effects on professional satisfaction. At the time of our study, "meaningful use" stood out as having particularly prominent effect on professional satisfaction. Physicians expressed frustration with the time, documentation, and lack of flexibility that meaningful-use rules imposed; their incongruity with clinical practice (especially outside primary care); and their contributions to the current state of EHR technology. An assessment of the burden of meaningful-use compliance on physicians and the readiness of EHR vendor community may be important as implementation proceeds.

- **Relationships with hospitals and health systems.** Within our sample, multiple practices had recently become hospital-owned or had established other types of affiliation with large delivery systems, but some expressed concerns about transitioning to these models of care. We found that values alignment between physicians and practice leadership was an important contributor to physician professional satisfaction and that a lack of control over operational, business, or managerial decisions affecting patient care could cause dissatisfaction. As physicians pursue employment, thoughtful engagement of physicians by including them in organizational decisions and leadership roles will be an important aspect of creating a satisfied physician team.

- **The need for additional payment methodologies.** Some physicians in our study described traditional fee-for-service payment as working fine. However, for many physicians (especially those in primary care), fee-for-service payment was a contributor to dissatisfaction, both due to the resulting time pressure and emphasis on the volume, rather than the quality, of patient care. These physicians are looking for additional or different payment approaches. Such approaches include, among others, subscription payments (including "concierge practice" models), bundled payments with hospitals, and a continuum of risk-bearing payment models designed to reward physicians for managing the appropriateness of the services their patients receive (whether provided directly by the responsible physician or by other providers). To the extent that physicians have knowledge of and access to a range of such payment choices and can choose those that fit their own practices the best, professional satisfaction seems likely to improve. However, several respondents described the transition between payment models as a period of potentially unstable physician incomes and practice finances, and physicians described income stability as being important to their professional satisfaction. Efforts to help physicians manage these transitions will be important to maintaining professional satisfaction and improving the likelihood that new payment models will have broad and successful uptake.

Implications for Health Policy and Systems

Many of the factors influencing physician professional satisfaction identified in this study are shared by professionals and workers in a wide variety of settings. Therefore, the same considerations that apply outside medicine—for example, fair treatment; responsive leadership; attention to work quantity, content, and pace—can serve as targets for policymakers and health delivery systems that seek to improve physician professional satisfaction. This may seem an obvious conclusion, but considering the typical toolkit used to influence physician behavior (regulations, payment rules, financial incentives, public reporting, and the threat of legal action), refocusing attention on the targets identified in this study may actually represent a substantial change of orientation for many participants in the U.S. health care system. This gives rise to a number of important questions that researchers, policymakers, and health care leaders need to answer going forward:

- Where will the knowledge base and resources needed for internal practice improvement come from? Many physician practices need help with managing change. Larger physician practices have begun to apply techniques, such as "lean," with success, but for the majority of physician practices, such interventions are out of reach without help. Are hospitals and health systems the only source for such practice improvement support?
- Will practice consolidation, especially the large-scale employment of physicians by hospitals and health systems, improve or detract from physician satisfaction over the longer term? If the latter, what will be the eventual outcome of having a potentially disenfranchised physician workforce? Some policymakers and organizations believe such a result can be prevented by the early development and spread of new models of physician-hospital integration and "comanagement."
- If income predictability and fairness contribute to physician practice satisfaction, will this be best achieved by fee-for-service payment in the future or by new and different payment methodologies? If the latter, what can be done to speed up such payment transformations while analyzing, adjusting, and strengthening or discarding these methodologies as more is learned about what really works and what does not? Where does the responsibility for this work rest, especially outside Medicare and Medicaid?
- Finally, we found that EHR usability represents a relatively new, unique, and vexing challenge to physician professional satisfaction. Few other service industries are exposed to universal and substantial incentives to adopt such a specific, highly regulated form of technology, which has, as our findings suggest, not yet matured. The current state of EHR technology appears to significantly worsen professional satisfaction for many physicians—sometimes in ways that raise concerns about effects on patient care.

   Physicians look forward to future EHRs that will solve current problems of data entry, difficult user interfaces, and information overload. Specific steps to hasten these technological advances are beyond the scope of this report. However, as a general principle, our findings suggest including improved EHR usability as a precondition for federal EHR certification. Until EHR usability improves dramatically, to the point where directly interacting with an EHR neither creates additional, excessive clerical work for physicians nor distracts from patient care, it may be advisable to remove regulatory and legal barriers to using other practice staff (e.g., scribes) to interact directly with EHRs, allowing physician more time to perform work that requires physicians' training.

   How, then, can we begin to turn the EHR "ocean liner," so that usability is improved, efficiency is improved by allowing more liberal use of the EHR by office staff, and meaningful-use standards develop over time at a pace more in line with the state of this distributed technology? Can a public-private partnership to do this be developed soon, before we see deterioration of or passive resistance to EHRs?

Answers to these questions, and successful interventions to address them, will do much to improve the professional satisfaction of the physician workforce and the quality, experience, and efficiency of patient care.

Advisory Committee Members

John E. Billi, MD
Professor of Internal Medicine, Medical Education and Associate Dean at the University of Michigan Medical School and Associate Vice President for Medical Affairs of the University of Michigan

Lawrence Casalino, MD, PhD
Chief of the Division of Outcomes and Effectiveness Research and Livingston Farrand Associate Professor of Public Health in the Department of Public Health at Weill Cornell Medical College

Carolyn Clancy, MD
Director of the Agency for Healthcare Research and Quality

Thomas Curry
Executive Director/CEO of the Washington State Medical Association

Edward Murphy, MD
Advisor at TowerBrook Capital Partners and a professor of Medicine at the Virginia Tech Carilion School of Medicine

Rick Wesslund, MBA
Founder and Chairman of BDC Advisors

Nicholas Wolter, MD
CEO of Billings Clinic

References

Adler-Milstein, J., D. W. Bates, and A. K. Jha, "Operational Health Information Exchanges Show Substantial Growth, but Long-Term Funding Remains a Concern," *Health Affairs,* Vol. 32, No. 8, August 2013, pp. 1486–1492. As of September 26, 2013:
http://www.ncbi.nlm.nih.gov/pubmed/23840051

Adler-Milstein, J., C. E. Green, and D. W. Bates, "A Survey Analysis Suggests That Electronic Health Records Will Yield Revenue Gains for Some Practices and Losses for Many," *Health Affairs,* Vol. 32, No. 3, March 2013, pp. 562–570. As of September 26, 2013:
http://www.ncbi.nlm.nih.gov/pubmed/23459736

An, P. G., J. S. Rabatin, L. B. Manwell, M. Linzer, R. L. Brown, and M. D. Schwartz, "Burden of Difficult Encounters in Primary Care: Data from the Minimizing Error, Maximizing Outcomes Study," *Archives of Internal Medicine,* Vol. 169, No. 4, February 23, 2009, pp. 410–414. As of September 26, 2013:
http://www.ncbi.nlm.nih.gov/pubmed/19237726

Armijo, D., C. McDonnell, and K. Werner, *Electronic Health Record Usability: Evaluation and Use Case Framework,* Rockville, MD: Agency for Healthcare Research and Quality, AHRQ Publication No. 09(10)-0091-1-EF, October 2009. As of September 26, 2013:
http://www.himss.org/files/HIMSSorg/content/files/Code%20119%20-%20EHR%20Usability_Evaluation%20and%20Use%20Case%20Framework_AHRQ.pdf

Boukus, E., A. Cassil, and A. S. O'Malley, "A Snapshot of U.S. Physicians: Key Findings from the 2008 Health Tracking Physician Survey," No. 35, 2009, pp. 1–11. As of September 26, 2013:
http://pubget.com/paper/19768851

Bradley, E. H., L. A. Curry, and K. J. Devers, "Qualitative Data Analysis for Health Services Research: Developing Taxonomy, Themes, and Theory," *Health Serv Res,* Vol. 42, No. 4, August 2007, pp. 1758–1772. As of September 26, 2013:
http://www.ncbi.nlm.nih.gov/pubmed/17286625

Buchbinder, S. B., M. Wilson, C. F. Melick, and N. R. Powe, "Estimates of Costs of Primary Care Physician Turnover," *Am J Manag Care,* Vol. 5, No. 11, November 1999, pp. 1431–1438. As of September 26, 2013:
http://www.ncbi.nlm.nih.gov/entrez/query.fcgi?cmd=Retrieve&db=PubMed&dopt=Citation&list_uids=10662416

———, "Primary Care Physician Job Satisfaction and Turnover," *Am J Manag Care,* Vol. 7, No. 7, July 2001, pp. 701–713. As of September 26, 2013:
http://www.ncbi.nlm.nih.gov/entrez/query.fcgi?cmd=Retrieve&db=PubMed&dopt=Citation&list_uids=11464428

Center for Studying Health System Change, "CTS Physician Surveys and the HSC 2008 Health Tracking Physician Survey," homepage, July 17, 2013. As of September 26, 2013:
http://www.hschange.com/index.cgi?data=04

Chen, P. G., L. A. Curry, M. Nunez-Smith, E. H. Bradley, and M. M. Desai, "Career Satisfaction in Primary Care: A Comparison of International and US Medical Graduates," *Journal of General Internal Medicine,* Vol. 27, No. 2, February 2012, pp. 147–152. As of September 26, 2013:
http://www.ncbi.nlm.nih.gov/pubmed/21866306

Cydulka, R. K., and R. Korte, "Career Satisfaction in Emergency Medicine: The ABEM Longitudinal Study of Emergency Physicians," *Ann Emerg Med,* Vol. 51, No. 6, 2008. As of September 26, 2013: http://pubget.com/paper/18395936

DeVoe, J., G. E. Fryer, Jr., A. Straub, J. McCann, and G. Fairbrother, "Congruent Satisfaction: Is There Geographic Correlation Between Patient and Physician Satisfaction?" *Med Care,* Vol. 45, No. 1, January 2007, pp. 88–94. As of September 26, 2013: http://www.ncbi.nlm.nih.gov/entrez/query.fcgi?cmd=Retrieve&db=PubMed&dopt=Citation&list_uids=17279025

DiMatteo, M. R., C. D. Sherbourne, R. D. Hays, L. Ordway, R. L. Kravitz, E. A. McGlynn, S. Kaplan, and W. H. Rogers, "Physicians' Characteristics Influence Patients' Adherence to Medical Treatment: Results from the Medical Outcomes Study," *Health Psychol,* Vol. 12, No. 2, 1993, pp. 93–102. As of September 26, 2013: http://pubget.com/paper/8500445

Dorsey, E. R., D. Jarjoura, and G. W. Rutecki, "Influence of Controllable Lifestyle on Recent Trends in Specialty Choice by US Medical Students," *JAMA,* Vol. 290, No. 9, September 3, 2003, pp. 1173–1178. As of September 26, 2013: http://www.ncbi.nlm.nih.gov/pubmed/12952999

El-Kareh, R., T. K. Gandhi, E. G. Poon, L. P. Newmark, J. Ungar, S. Lipsitz, and T. D. Sequist, "Trends in Primary Care Clinician Perceptions of a New Electronic Health Record," *J Gen Intern Med,* Vol. 24, No. 4, April 2009, pp. 464–468. As of September 26, 2013: http://www.ncbi.nlm.nih.gov/pubmed/19156468

Fernandopulle, R., and N. Patel, "How the Electronic Health Record Did Not Measure Up to the Demands of Our Medical Home Practice," *Health Affairs,* Vol. 29, No. 4, April 2010, pp. 622–628. As of September 26, 2013: http://www.ncbi.nlm.nih.gov/pubmed/20368591

Frank, E., J. E. McMurray, M. Linzer, and L. Elon, "Career Satisfaction of US Women Physicians: Results from the Women Physicians' Health Study, Society of General Internal Medicine Career Satisfaction Study Group," *Arch Intern Med,* Vol. 159, No. 13, July 12, 1999, pp. 1417–1426. As of September 26, 2013: http://www.ncbi.nlm.nih.gov/entrez/query.fcgi?cmd=Retrieve&db=PubMed&dopt=Citation&list_uids=10399893

Friedberg, M. W., "The Potential Impact of the Medical Home on Job Satisfaction in Primary Care," *Archives of Internal Medicine,* Vol. 172, No. 1, January 9, 2012, pp. 31–32. As of September 26, 2013: http://www.ncbi.nlm.nih.gov/pubmed/22232144

Friedberg, M. W., D. G. Safran, K. L. Coltin, M. Dresser, and E. C. Schneider, "Readiness for the Patient-Centered Medical Home: Structural Capabilities of Massachusetts Primary Care Practices," *J Gen Intern Med,* Vol. 24, No. 2, February 2009, pp. 162–169.

Grembowski, D., D. Paschane, P. Diehr, W. Katon, D. Martin, and D. L. Patrick, "Managed Care, Physician Job Satisfaction, and the Quality of Primary Care," *Journal of General Internal Medicine,* Vol. 20, No. 3, March 2005, pp. 271–277. As of September 26, 2013: http://www.ncbi.nlm.nih.gov/pubmed/15836532

Grembowski, D., C. M. Ulrich, D. Paschane, P. Diehr, W. Katon, D. Martin, D. L. Patrick, and C. Velicer, "Managed Care and Primary Physician Satisfaction," *Journal of the American Board of Family Practice/ American Board of Family Practice,* Vol. 16, No. 5, September–October 2003, pp. 383–393. As of September 26, 2013: http://www.ncbi.nlm.nih.gov/pubmed/14645328

Haas, J. S., E. F. Cook, A. L. Puopolo, H. R. Burstin, P. D. Cleary, and T. A. Brennan, "Is the Professional Satisfaction of General Internists Associated with Patient Satisfaction?" *J Gen Intern Med,* Vol. 15, No. 2, February 2000, pp. 122–128. As of September 26, 2013: http://www.ncbi.nlm.nih.gov/entrez/query.fcgi?cmd=Retrieve&db=PubMed&dopt=Citation&list_uids=10672116

Hadley, J., and J. M. Mitchell, "Effects of HMO Market Penetration on Physicians' Work Effort and Satisfaction," *Health Affairs,* Vol. 16, No. 6, November–December 1997, pp. 99–111. As of September 26, 2013:
http://www.ncbi.nlm.nih.gov/pubmed/9444813

Hill, C. E., S. Knox, B. J. Thompson, E. N. Williams, S. A. Hess, and N. Ladany, "Consensual Qualitative Research: An Update," *Journal of Counseling Psychology,* Vol. 52, No. 2, April 2005, pp. 196–205.

Hirschtick, R. E., "A Piece of My Mind: Copy-and-Paste," *JAMA,* Vol. 295, No. 20, May 24, 2006, pp. 2335–2336. As of September 26, 2013:
http://www.ncbi.nlm.nih.gov/pubmed/16720812

Institute of Medicine, *Health IT and Patient Safety: Building Safer Systems for Better Care,* Washington, D.C., 2012.

Jaen, C. R., B. F. Crabtree, R. F. Palmer, R. L. Ferrer, P. A. Nutting, W. L. Miller, E. E. Stewart, R. Wood, M. Davila, and K. C. Stange, "Methods for Evaluating Practice Change Toward a Patient-Centered Medical Home," *Ann Fam Med,* Vol. 8, Suppl. 1, May 1, 2010, 2010, pp. S9–20. As of September 26, 2013:
http://www.annfammed.org/cgi/content/abstract/8/Suppl_1/S9

Johnson, C. W., "Why Did That Happen? Exploring the Proliferation of Barely Usable Software in Healthcare Systems," *Qual Saf Health Care,* Vol. 15, Suppl. 1, December 2006, pp. i76–81. As of September 26, 2013:
http://www.ncbi.nlm.nih.gov/pubmed/17142614

Karsh, B. T., J. W. Beasley, and R. L. Brown, "Employed Family Physician Satisfaction and Commitment to Their Practice, Work Group, and Health Care Organization," *Health Services Research,* Vol. 45, No. 2, April 2010, pp. 457–475. As of September 26, 2013:
http://www.ncbi.nlm.nih.gov/pubmed/20070386

Kemper, P., D. Blumenthal, J. M. Corrigan, P. J. Cunningham, S. M. Felt, J. M. Grossman, L. T. Kohn, C. E. Metcalf, R. F. St. Peter, R. C. Strouse, and P. B. Ginsburg, "The Design of the Community Tracking Study: A Longitudinal Study of Health System Change and Its Effects on People," *Inquiry : A Journal of Medical Care Organization, Provision and Financing,* Vol. 33, No. 2, Summer 1996, pp. 195–206. As of September 26, 2013:
http://www.ncbi.nlm.nih.gov/pubmed/8675282

Konrad, T. R., E. S. Williams, M. Linzer, J. McMurray, D. E. Pathman, M. Gerrity, M. D. Schwartz, W. E. Scheckler, J. Van Kirk, E. Rhodes, and J. Douglas, "Measuring Physician Job Satisfaction in a Changing Workplace and a Challenging Environment," SGIM Career Satisfaction Study Group, Society of General Internal Medicine, *Med Care,* Vol. 37, No. 11, November 1999, pp. 1174–1182. As of September 26, 2013:
http://www.ncbi.nlm.nih.gov/entrez/query.fcgi?cmd=Retrieve&db=PubMed&dopt=Citation&list_uids=10549620

Koppel, R., "Is Healthcare Information Technology Based on Evidence?" *Yearb Med Inform,* Vol. 8, No. 1, 2013, pp. 7–12. As of September 26, 2013:
http://www.ncbi.nlm.nih.gov/pubmed/23974542

Koppel, R., J. P. Metlay, A. Cohen, B. Abaluck, A. R. Localio, S. E. Kimmel, and B. L. Strom, "Role of Computerized Physician Order Entry Systems in Facilitating Medication Errors," *JAMA,* Vol. 293, No. 10, March 9, 2005, pp. 1197–1203. As of September 26, 2013:
http://www.ncbi.nlm.nih.gov/pubmed/15755942

Kuusio, H., T. Heponiemi, A. M. Aalto, T. Sinervo, and M. Elovainio, "Differences in Well-Being Between GPs, Medical Specialists, and Private Physicians: The Role of Psychosocial Factors," *Health Services Research,* Vol. 47, No. 1 Pt. 1, February 2012, pp. 68–85. As of September 26, 2013:
http://www.ncbi.nlm.nih.gov/pubmed/22091688

Kvale, Steinar, *Interviews: An Introduction to Qualitative Research Interviewing,* Thousand Oaks, CA: Sage Publications, 1996.

Landon, B. E., R. Aseltine, Jr., J. A. Shaul, Y. Miller, B. A. Auerbach, and P. D. Cleary, "Evolving Dissatisfaction Among Primary Care Physicians," *Am J Manag Care,* Vol. 8, No. 10, October 2002, pp. 890–901. As of September 26, 2013:
http://www.ncbi.nlm.nih.gov/entrez/query.fcgi?cmd=Retrieve&db=PubMed&dopt=Citation&list_uids=12395957

Landon, B. E., J. Reschovsky, and D. Blumenthal, "Changes in Career Satisfaction Among Primary Care and Specialist Physicians, 1997–2001," *JAMA,* Vol. 289, No. 4, January 22–29, 2003, pp. 442–449. As of September 26, 2013:
http://www.ncbi.nlm.nih.gov/entrez/query.fcgi?cmd=Retrieve&db=PubMed&dopt=Citation&list_uids=12533123

Landon, B. E., J. D. Reschovsky, H. H. Pham, and D. Blumenthal, "Leaving Medicine: The Consequences of Physician Dissatisfaction," *Med Care,* Vol. 44, No. 3, March 2006, pp. 234–242. As of September 26, 2013:
http://www.ncbi.nlm.nih.gov/entrez/query.fcgi?cmd=Retrieve&db=PubMed&dopt=Citation&list_uids=16501394

Leigh, J. P., R. L. Kravitz, M. Schembri, S. J. Samuels, and S. Mobley, "Physician Career Satisfaction Across Specialties," *Arch Intern Med,* Vol. 162, No. 14, July 22, 2002, pp. 1577–1584. As of September 26, 2013:
http://www.ncbi.nlm.nih.gov/entrez/query.fcgi?cmd=Retrieve&db=PubMed&dopt=Citation&list_uids=12123400

Leigh, J. P., D. J. Tancredi, and R. L. Kravitz, "Physician Career Satisfaction Within Specialties," *BMC Health Serv Res,* Vol. 9, 2009, p. 166. As of September 26, 2013:
http://www.ncbi.nlm.nih.gov/entrez/query.fcgi?cmd=Retrieve&db=PubMed&dopt=Citation&list_uids=19758454

Lewis, J. M., F. D. Barnhart, B. L. Howard, D. I. Carson, and E. P. Nace, "Work Satisfaction in the Lives of Physicians," *Tex Med,* Vol. 89, No. 2, February 1993a, pp. 54–61. As of September 26, 2013:
http://www.ncbi.nlm.nih.gov/entrez/query.fcgi?cmd=Retrieve&db=PubMed&dopt=Citation&list_uids=8430387

———, "Work Stress in the Lives of Physicians," *Tex Med,* Vol. 89, No. 2, February 1993b, pp. 62–67. As of September 26, 2013:
http://www.ncbi.nlm.nih.gov/entrez/query.fcgi?cmd=Retrieve&db=PubMed&dopt=Citation&list_uids=8430388

Lewis, S. E., R. S. Nocon, H. Tang, S. Y. Park, A. M. Vable, L. P. Casalino, E. S. Huang, M. T. Quinn, D. L. Burnet, W. T. Summerfelt, J. M. Birnberg, and M. H. Chin, "Patient-Centered Medical Home Characteristics and Staff Morale in Safety Net Clinics," *Arch Intern Med,* Vol. 172, No. 1, January 9, 2012a, pp. 23–31. As of September 26, 2013:
http://www.ncbi.nlm.nih.gov/pubmed/22232143

Liang, K. Y., and S. Zeger, "Longitudinal Data Analysis Using Generalized Linear Models," *Biometrika,* Vol. 73, 1986, pp. 13–22.

Linn, L. S., R. H. Brook, V. A. Clark, A. R. Davies, A. Fink, and J. Kosecoff, "Physician and Patient Satisfaction as Factors Related to the Organization of Internal Medicine Group Practices," *Med Care,* Vol. 23, No. 10, October 1985, pp. 1171–1178. As of September 26, 2013:
http://www.ncbi.nlm.nih.gov/entrez/query.fcgi?cmd=Retrieve&db=PubMed&dopt=Citation&list_uids=4058071

Linn, L. S., R. H. Brook, V. A. Clark, A. R. Davies, A. Fink, J. Kosecoff, and P. Salisbury, "Work Satisfaction and Career Aspirations of Internists Working in Teaching Hospital Group Practices," *J Gen Intern Med,* Vol. 1, No. 2, March–April, 1986, pp. 104–108. As of September 26, 2013:
http://www.ncbi.nlm.nih.gov/entrez/query.fcgi?cmd=Retrieve&db=PubMed&dopt=Citation&list_uids=3772572

Linn, L. S., J. Yager, D. Cope, and B. Leake, "Health Status, Job Satisfaction, Job Stress, and Life Satisfaction Among Academic and Clinical Faculty," *JAMA,* Vol. 254, No. 19, November 15, 1985, pp. 2775–2782. As of September 26, 2013:
http://www.ncbi.nlm.nih.gov/entrez/query.fcgi?cmd=Retrieve&db=PubMed&dopt=Citation&list_uids=4057485

Linzer, M., M. Gerrity, J. A. Douglas, J. E. McMurray, E. S. Williams, and T. R. Konrad, "Physician Stress: Results from the Physician Worklife Study," *Stress Health,* Vol. 18, No. 1, 2002, pp. 37–42. As of September 26, 2013:
http://dx.doi.org/10.1002/smi.917

Linzer, M., T. R. Konrad, J. Douglas, J. E. McMurray, D. E. Pathman, E. S. Williams, M. D. Schwartz, M. Gerrity, W. Scheckler, J. A. Bigby, and E. Rhodes, "Managed Care, Time Pressure, and Physician Job Satisfaction: Results from the Physician Worklife Study," *J Gen Intern Med,* Vol. 15, No. 7, July 2000, pp. 441–450. As of September 26, 2013:
http://www.ncbi.nlm.nih.gov/entrez/query.fcgi?cmd=Retrieve&db=PubMed&dopt=Citation&list_uids=10940129

Linzer, M., L. B. Manwell, E. S. Williams, J. A. Bobula, R. L. Brown, A. B. Varkey, B. Man, J. E. McMurray, A. Maguire, B. Horner-Ibler, and M. D. Schwartz, "Working Conditions in Primary Care: Physician Reactions and Care Quality," *Ann Intern Med,* Vol. 151, No. 1, July 7, 2009, pp. 28–36, W26–29.

Love, J. S., A. Wright, S. R. Simon, C. A. Jenter, C. S. Soran, L. A. Volk, D. W. Bates, and E. G. Poon, "Are Physicians' Perceptions of Healthcare Quality and Practice Satisfaction Affected by Errors Associated with Electronic Health Record Use?" *J Am Med Inform Assoc,* Vol. 19, No. 4, July–August 2012, pp. 610–614. As of September 26, 2013:
http://www.ncbi.nlm.nih.gov/pubmed/22199017

McConnell, K. J., R. C. Lindrooth, D. R. Wholey, T. M. Maddox, and N. Bloom, "Management Practices and the Quality of Care in Cardiac Units," *JAMA Intern Med,* Vol. 173, No. 8, Apr 22, 2013, pp. 684–692. As of September 26, 2013:
http://www.ncbi.nlm.nih.gov/pubmed/23552986

Menachemi, N., T. L. Powers, and R. G. Brooks, "The Role of Information Technology Usage in Physician Practice Satisfaction," *Health Care Management Review,* Vol. 34, No. 4, October–December 2009, pp. 364–371. As of September 26, 2013:
http://www.ncbi.nlm.nih.gov/pubmed/19858921

Middleton, B., M. Bloomrosen, M. A. Dente, B. Hashmat, R. Koppel, J. M. Overhage, T. H. Payne, S. T. Rosenbloom, C. Weaver, and J. Zhang, "Enhancing Patient Safety and Quality of Care by Improving the Usability of Electronic Health Record Systems: Recommendations from AMIA," *J Am Med Inform Assoc,* Vol. 20, No. e1, June 2013, pp. e2–8. As of September 26, 2013:
http://www.ncbi.nlm.nih.gov/pubmed/23355463

Moran-Ellis, Jo, Victoria D. Alexander, Ann Cronin, Mary Dickinson, Jane Fielding, Judith Sleney, and Hilary Thomas, "Triangulation and Integration: Processes, Claims and Implications," *Qualitative Research,* Vol. 6, No. 1, February 1, 2006, pp. 45–59. As of September 26, 2013:
http://qrj.sagepub.com/content/6/1/45.abstract

Movassaghi, H., and D. Kindig, "Medical Practice and Satisfaction of Physicians in Sparsely Populated Rural Counties of the United States: Results of a 1988 Survey," *J Rural Health,* Vol. 5, No. 2, April 1989, pp. 125–136. As of September 26, 2013:
http://www.ncbi.nlm.nih.gov/entrez/query.fcgi?cmd=Retrieve&db=PubMed&dopt=Citation&list_uids=10294462

O'Cathain, A., E. Murphy, and J. Nicholl, "Three Techniques for Integrating Data in Mixed Methods Studies," *BMJ,* Vol. 341, 2010, p. c4587. As of September 26, 2013:
http://www.ncbi.nlm.nih.gov/pubmed/20851841

O'Malley, A. S., J. M. Grossman, G. R. Cohen, N. M. Kemper, and H. H. Pham, "Are Electronic Medical Records Helpful for Care Coordination? Experiences of Physician Practices," *J Gen Intern Med,* Vol. 25, No. 3, March 2010, pp. 177–185. As of September 26, 2013:
http://www.ncbi.nlm.nih.gov/pubmed/20033621

Pagan, J. A., L. Balasubramanian, and M. V. Pauly, "Physicians' Career Satisfaction, Quality of Care and Patients' Trust: The Role of Community Uninsurance," *Health Econ Policy Law,* Vol. 2, Pt. 4, October 2007, pp. 347–362. As of September 26, 2013:
http://www.ncbi.nlm.nih.gov/entrez/query.fcgi?cmd=Retrieve&db=PubMed&dopt=Citation&list_uids=18634638

The Physicians Foundation, *A Survey of America's Physicians: Practice Patterns and Perspectives*, September 2012. As of September 26, 2013:
http://www.physiciansfoundation.org/uploads/default/Physicians_Foundation_2012_Biennial_Survey.pdf

Podsakoff, P. M., S. B. MacKenzie, J. Y. Lee, and N. P. Podsakoff, "Common Method Biases in Behavioral Research: A Critical Review of the Literature and Recommended Remedies," *J Appl Psychol,* Vol. 88, No. 5, October 2003, pp. 879–903. As of September 26, 2013:
http://www.ncbi.nlm.nih.gov/pubmed/14516251

Quinn, M. A., A. Wilcox, E. J. Orav, D. W. Bates, and S. R. Simon, "The Relationship Between Perceived Practice Quality and Quality Improvement Activities and Physician Practice Dissatisfaction, Professional Isolation, and Work-Life Stress," *Medical Care,* Vol. 47, No. 8, August 2009, pp. 924–928. As of September 26, 2013:
http://www.ncbi.nlm.nih.gov/pubmed/19543122

Reid, R. J., K. Coleman, E. A. Johnson, P. A. Fishman, C. Hsu, M. P. Soman, C. E. Trescott, M. Erikson, and E. B. Larson, "The Group Health Medical Home at Year Two: Cost Savings, Higher Patient Satisfaction, and Less Burnout for Providers," *Health Affairs,* Vol. 29, No. 5, May 2010, pp. 835–843. As of September 26, 2013:
http://www.ncbi.nlm.nih.gov/pubmed/20439869

Scheier, M. F., C. S. Carver, and M. W. Bridges, "Distinguishing Optimism from Aneuroticism (and Trait Anxiety, Self-Mastery, and Self-Esteem): A Reevaluation of the Life Orientation Test," *J Pers Soc Psychol,* Vol. 67, No. 6, December 1994, pp. 1063–1078. As of September 26, 2013:
http://www.ncbi.nlm.nih.gov/pubmed/7815302

Sinsky, C. A., R. Willard-Grace, A. M. Schutzbank, T. A. Sinsky, D. Margolius, and T. Bodenheimer, "In Search of Joy in Practice: A Report of 23 High-Functioning Primary Care Practices," *Annals of Family Medicine,* Vol. 11, No. 3, May–June 2013, pp. 272–278. As of September 26, 2013:
http://www.ncbi.nlm.nih.gov/pubmed/23690328

Stoddard, J. J., J. L. Hargraves, M. Reed, and A. Vratil, "Managed Care, Professional Autonomy, and Income: Effects on Physician Career Satisfaction," *J Gen Intern Med,* Vol. 16, No. 10, October 2001, pp. 675–684. As of September 26, 2013:
http://www.ncbi.nlm.nih.gov/entrez/query.fcgi?cmd=Retrieve&db=PubMed&dopt=Citation&list_uids=11679035

Warren, M. G., R. Weitz, and S. Kulis, "Physician Satisfaction in a Changing Health Care Environment: The Impact of Challenges to Professional Autonomy, Authority, and Dominance," *J Health Soc Behav,* Vol. 39, No. 4, December 1998, pp. 356–367. As of September 26, 2013:
http://www.ncbi.nlm.nih.gov/entrez/query.fcgi?cmd=Retrieve&db=PubMed&dopt=Citation&list_uids=9919857

Wetterneck, T. B., M. Linzer, J. E. McMurray, J. Douglas, M. D. Schwartz, J. Bigby, M. S. Gerrity, D. E. Pathman, D. Karlson, and E. Rhodes, "Worklife and Satisfaction of General Internists," *Archives of Internal Medicine,* Vol. 162, No. 6, March 25, 2002, pp. 649–656. As of September 26, 2013:
http://www.ncbi.nlm.nih.gov/pubmed/11911718

Williams, E. S., T. R. Konrad, M. Linzer, J. McMurray, D. E. Pathman, M. Gerrity, M. D. Schwartz, W. E. Scheckler, J. Van Kirk, E. Rhodes, and J. Douglas, "Refining the Measurement of Physician Job Satisfaction: Results from the Physician Worklife Survey," SGIM Career Satisfaction Study Group, Society of General Internal Medicine, *Med Care,* Vol. 37, No. 11, November 1999, pp. 1140–1154. As of September 26, 2013:
http://www.ncbi.nlm.nih.gov/entrez/query.fcgi?cmd=Retrieve&db=PubMed&dopt=Citation&list_uids=10549616

Zeger, S. L., and K. Y. Liang, "Longitudinal Data Analysis for Discrete and Continuous Outcomes," *Biometrics,* Vol. 42, No. 1, March 1986, pp. 121–130.